To Bill —

With Much Appreciation

For The Book Club's

Contribution to my

own Health and

Well Being.

8-26-85

Improving Rural Health
Initiatives of an
Academic Medical Center

Thomas Allen Bruce, M.D.
Dean, College of Medicine
University of Arkansas for Medical Sciences

W. Richard Norton
Director, Office of Research
Division of Rural Medical Development
University of Arkansas for Medical Sciences

Rose Publishing Company
Little Rock, Arkansas

Bruce, Thomas.
    Improving rural health: initiatives of an academic
medical center.

    Bibliography: p. 188
    1. Rural health services—Arkansas.   2. Medicine, Rural—
Arkansas.   3. University of Arkansas for Medical Sciences.
I. Norton, Richard.   II. Title.

RA771.6.A7   362.10425   84-51672
ISBN 0-914546-53-8

Dedication

This book is dedicated to the faculty of the College of Medicine, University of Arkansas for Medical Sciences (members of the Medical College Physicians Group), who through contributions to the Dean's Development Fund have provided the primary financial sustenance for the Rural Medical Development Program during the past ten years. These faculty members have lent their wisdom, counsel and enthusiastic support for the outreach efforts which have contributed so importantly to the improvements in rural medical care.

Acknowledgements

In 1976 the Winthrop Rockefeller Foundation provided a grant to the College of Medicine, University of Arkansas for Medical Sciences, which initiated the Rural Medical Research Program. Tom McRae and Bob Nash of the Foundation and other members of the staff have been interested and supportive in the years which have followed and have given freely of their time and counsel. The editors wish also to acknowledge the help of Ted Williams and his associates at Winrock International on Petit Jean Mountain for their hospitality and thoughtfulness at the planning retreats of the Rural Medical Development Program staff, as well as the advice they tendered on the advantages and disadvantages in developing a regional, national or international center on rural health.

For the outstanding participation of the Arkansas practicing physicians, as well as that of the medical students and the house-staff, in answering the endless questionnaires, we will be perpetually grateful. They also involved themselves wholeheartedly in the assorted experimental efforts which were designed to make improvements in rural medical care. Our colleagues in the Arkansas Medical Society likewise have been genuinely cooperative at every turn; Ken LaMastus deserves special mention for his congenial helpfulness.

Our friends at the main campus of the University of Arkansas in Fayetteville deserve much praise for their time and effort in support of the Program. In particular, Reed Greenwood from the Rehabilitation Education and Research faculty was a valuable resource in serving as the coordinator for several planning meetings, and Don Voth in Rural Sociology and Mary Jo Schneider in Anthropology were involved in the conceptual framework of the medical studies.

In Little Rock, Forrest Pollard at the University of Arkansas Industrial Research and Extension Center always was resourceful in supplying needed Arkansas data. We are also indebted to the

University of Arkansas Cooperative Extension Service which, through their Health Education staff and the 75 county-level offices throughout the state, worked so diligently in our behalf.

Jim Bernstein of the North Carolina Office of Rural Health Services has been a valuable ally and consultant in several phases of the Arkansas work. He and his staff went to great effort to show us some of the rural health clinics developed through his Office, and in several visits to Arkansas he has reviewed the plans and offered helpful suggestions about the directions for our own Program.

We offer our gratitude to Bernal Green in the U.S. Department of Agriculture for the insight and frequent encouragement he provided for the community development and health education activities. Orson Berry and Gary Jones at the Arkansas Department of Health have been involved on a continuing basis, and Ben Saltzman, the present Director of the Department, has been an integral and critical part of these efforts from the beginning. We also are grateful for the thoughtful suggestions of Linda Bilheimer, who served jointly as a member of the medical faculty and as the Health Economist for the Health Department. The state health planning committees and the health systems agencies deserve recognition for their cooperation.

Finally, the editors wish to express special appreciation to Judy Smith, Suzanne Hicks and Kathryn Young for their dogged assistance, patience and fortitude in the preparation of this volume.

Contents

Foreword

In 1972 Arkansas was experiencing all of the changes in medical practice that were occurring throughout the country. Rural communities were without physicians, an abundance of specialists had settled in the major city of Little Rock, a sense of indifference on the part of the medical school was perceived by the general public and elected leaders, a second medical school emphasizing family medicine was being considered and, of most concern, mortality and morbidity tables were beginning to show the negative effect that absence of medical care can have on both the duration and quality of life.

A decade later a dramatic reversal had occurred. In fact, Arkansas had developed a mature modular health education network, was now facing a physician surplus, and had changed mortality and morbidity tables to above the average in virtually every category.

This is an important book, both conceptually and as an instruction manual on "How To Do It." Although every step is not applicable to other regions, the majority of the information is transferable and can serve as guidelines that should be considered in planning a comprehensive rural health program.

The energy and the commitment of the medical school faculty and administration cannot be overemphasized. The conflicting priorities of academic life forced many compromises. It is noteworthy that educational standards and achievement as measured by national examinations, etc. were maintained. Biomedical research may have suffered slightly and efforts are now underway to expand these programs. But, in balance, the University of Arkansas Medical College thrived, protected and expanded the tradition of education, service and research upon which our academic institutions are founded.

Harry P. Ward, M.D.
Chancellor, University of Arkansas for Medical Sciences

Preface

There is, in the mid-1980's, a growing consensus that the doctor shortage is behind us, that medical schools are educating plenty of physicians for the future. There even is talk in some quarters about a physician surplus, with statements of general concern that the nation should begin to cut back on its medical training programs.

Rural America doesn't see it quite that way. Things are better, yes, but there is still a significant gap between what is available and what is needed or desired. The authors of the 1980 Summary Report of the Graduate Medical Education National Advisory Committee, generally called the GMENAC Report, didn't see the big new supply of physicians as the final solution to future medical care needs either:

> There will be TOO MANY physicians in 1990. There will be substantial IMBALANCES in some specialties. There will continue to be a marked UNEVENNESS in the geographic distribution of physicians. The country may be training TOO MANY nonphysician providers for 1990. The factors influencing specialty choice are COMPLEX. The actual cost of graduate medical education is UNKNOWN. Economic motivation in specialty and geographic choice is UNCERTAIN.

The problem of maldistribution of people and resources is not new to rural communities. The problem of inadequate health resources is no worse than, as an example, the inadequacies in the public schools, the unavailability of important social support services and poor streets and roads. What is different in the health arena is that there is now a better understanding of the components of the problem and the issues that are needed to make good health care more accessible to all.

Health is an ideal, a vision. *Rural* health, in the mind's eye, conjures up scenes of apple cheeks, rugged physical fitness and emotional serenity in a rustic, pastoral setting. What exists in actuality is a surprisingly heterogeneous cluster of individuals in communities of various sizes, *some* of whom may be healthy. All too many, unfortunately, have an assortment of ailments or frequent illnesses. Many rural citizens are elderly and are subject to the limitations and special health problems of older people. Numerous others, for reasons of poverty and isolation and ignorance of the options, have difficulty in gaining access to health/medical care.

This book will focus on one medical school's efforts to understand and deal with the significant issues of rural health and medical services. It is not intended to be so much an anthology or archival record as it is a guide for other schools, professional societies, state legislative bodies and community action groups who are interested in improvements in rural medical care.

If there is one lesson to be learned from the Arkansas experience over the past ten years, it is that medical education and medical practice are not islands. Medical care is an integral part of the community in which it occurs. The physician "product" of the medical school must fit easily and well into the community "receptor site" or no functional union occurs; this is such a fundamental concept that it is easily overlooked by both parties.

Melding these two entities is especially difficult because medical care technology and community development are always in a state of flux. Misconceptions and preconceived ideas handicap both the doctor interested in rural practice and the small community interested in recruiting a new physician. The interplay between these two forces serves as the central theme which binds the individual chapters of this book into a cohesive document. It is our hope that the delineation of these rural medical studies and their conclusions will provide new insight into the issues at play and will stimulate a greater commitment for change in those who seek worldwide improvements in rural health.

T.A.B.
W.R.N.

God made the country,
and man made the town.

. . . William Cowper
The Task, Book I, 1.749.

Section I. The Rural Problem

It is impossible to deal with any matter of concern in a logical or effective manner without defining the precise nature of the problem and the specific components which, when addressed, might lead to resolution of the difficulty. As with so many other biological and social issues, the various aspects of rural health and of better rural medical care are enormously complex and not prone to easy solution.

Staff members in the College of Medicine discovered quite early some of the complexities to be faced. Aware of the growing public perception that the school's educational thrust was not addressing the immediate needs of the state's communities, the College in the early 1970's agreed to help enlist some of its own graduates in service to the neediest areas. It soon became apparent that the professors and medical school officials also were not effective in rural recruitment; in the few instances of seeming success the solution all too often was short-lived. Something more had to be done; some very basic and fundamental issues were not being addressed.

The five chapters which follow delineate some of the studies that were initiated to define more clearly the nature of the problem. It should be understood that we were a *medical* school and therefore singularly focused on the "doctor" issues. The initial studies looked primarily at the characteristics of the physicians, their attitudes, and the issues which seemed to shape their thoughts and behavior about rural practice. Only later did we begin to study some of the more obvious community variables of the problem, and then without getting into the more specific sociological issues which deal with total community development.

Chapter 1 sets the stage for the research studies by providing some of the background and early research that led to the creation of a Division of Rural Development Programs in the College. Chapter 2 presents in an abbreviated manner the first survey of all practicing physicians in Arkansas. That survey included demographic information, educational background and the sequence of each doctor's practice experiences. Chapter 3 outlines the results of the second general survey, including each physician's reasons for choosing an urban or rural practice and the assessment of any moves from one town to another. Chapter 4 reports serial surveys on the attitudes about specialty career and location decisions among medical students and housestaff. Finally, Chapter 5 compares some of the characteristics of "successful" and "unsuccessful" rural towns in the state.

Chapter 1
Reasons for Concern

by Thomas Allen Bruce, M.D.

It is my belief, Watson, founded on my experience, that the lowest and vilest alleys of London do not present a more dreadful record of sin than does the smiling and beautiful countryside.

... Sir Arthur Conan Doyle, "The Adventure of the Copper Beeches," *Adventures of Sherlock Holmes.*

Health professionals education represents one of the South's major successes . . . [but] despite increases in the overall supply . . . serious problems of distribution of professionals to geographic, subspecialty, and public service areas of need continue, except for those situations in which carefully coordinated strategies have been directed to specific problems.

... Southern Regional Education Board, 1983.

It is not unusual for a medical school to be interested in the delivery of medical care in rural areas; most medical schools in America, in fact, have active programs to study and evaluate the availability and quality of care in underserved areas. It is most unusual, on the other hand, for a medical school to go to the lengths of involvement seen in Arkansas from 1974 through 1983, where a sizable portion of the entire school's efforts and resources were devoted to improvements in rural medical care.

On September 13, 1972, then-Governor Dale Bumpers authorized the design of a new State Health Plan by a select group of state health professionals, serving as an ad hoc Committee. In a January 1973 report, the Committee defined two basic problems:

One problem is *health manpower*. Arkansas has both *shortages* of primary care personnel as well as *maldistribution* of existing personnel. The result is that no area of the State can claim to have sufficient personnel to meet the health care needs of all its population and a significant number of areas have no personnel at all in many critical health occupations .... The urban areas in the State cannot be said to have enough personnel for the populations they are expected to serve. The more serious shortages in rural areas cause population outside the logical service areas of urban centers to seek care from these already overtaxed community resources.

A second problem arises from the *inability of a sizeable portion of Arkansas' population to have ready access to primary care services*. This problem is related to the manpower problem as well as an inability to pay for care and the lack of actual physical facilities for rendering care in many communities. Almost 23% of Arkansas families ... live in poverty .. with an average annual family income of $1,947.

Six priorities were established by the Committee:

1. Establish Area Health Education Centers ... to develop training and continuing education programs for primary health service personnel and for community service manpower.
2. Develop training programs for physician extenders ....
3. Increase the capabilities of the University of Arkansas Medical Center to meet needs ... through: 1) an increase in the production of family practitioners ... and 2) an in-out WATS consultation system.
4. Develop and implement an Emergency Medical Services [program] ....
5. Increase the capabilities of the Arkansas Health Department for meeting primary health care needs through: 1) establishment of District Health Offices; 2) provision of additional nurses, sanitarians, and health educators in scarcity areas; 3) development of Ambulatory Centers in scarcity areas; 4) expansion of ... dental care and transportation ....; and 5) telephone access system.
6. Extend the scope of Title XIX to include reimbursement for: 1) medical assistance to the medically needy; 2) prescription drugs; 3) family planning; 4) home health services; 5) clinic services, and 6) nursing home services for clients under 21.

The governor responded to this report by putting together a state-wide coalition of leading citizens who in turn worked with key legislative groups to provide special funds to implement these six major recommendations. The College of Medicine in late 1973 found itself holding an official mandate to proceed with carrying out a major section of the plan.

An overriding mission was formulated for the medical school at a faculty planning retreat in 1974: training the numbers and types of physicians to meet the medical needs of Arkansas. Because this basically is a rural state, the plan called for academic attention to unresolved rural health issues and it set up an action-oriented program for medical school intervention.

The ramifications of this innocuous-sounding plan were, in fact, to be profound. The classical functions of a medical school have been to teach the scientific basis for disease and to educate new physicians in effective ways to treat those who are ill. Promoting specific medical career specialties and a geographic (rural) practice site for graduates, plus defining the particular educational support systems which would be needed to achieve these goals—all these were significant changes from this classical tradition. Moreover, when the mission was broadened still further to train not only the physicians, but also the rural towns in which doctors were to locate, a major departure had emerged from the comfortable medical school role of the previous hundred years.

It became apparent that in order to accomplish this mission, the most pressing need was for reliable information. The College could ill afford to make decisions of the magnitude that seemed necessary without accurate data. In 1975 the Office of Research in the Division of Rural Medical Development was established to develop such information. The hope was that the data would lead to well-informed decisions which would address many of the problems identified.

Immediately after the Office was established, discussions began with representatives of the Winthrop Rockefeller Foundation, based in Arkansas, about financial support to conduct a series of field surveys designed to provide the information needed. The concept was broadened at the request of the Foundation to include actions which the University could implement immediately to help alleviate several of the more pressing problems. The project was granted matching funds by the Foundation in mid-1976, with the following statement of purpose:

> ... to upgrade the health of the rural citizens of Arkansas by addressing the problem of adequate numbers of properly trained physicians in the small towns of the state.

5

We propose to investigate in detail some preliminary findings which indicate an anomalous Arkansas phenomenon, in which seemingly adequate numbers of physicians are locating in rural Arkansas communities after graduation from medical college, following which large numbers (approximately half) leave to relocate elsewhere during the first two years ... It is our intent to analyze the factors involved in this shift and to develop problem-solving remedial approaches which might be taken by the College of Medicine.

The Bottom Line—Not Enough Doctors

In the early 1970's an analysis of the nation's health manpower was made by the U.S. Department of Health, Education, and Welfare (DHEW). Arkansas was found to have one of the lowest physician-population ratios in the United States and to have 74 of her 75 counties "medically underserved" according to a standard formula. Indeed, the only county in the state that was NOT medically underserved was Sebastian County near the Oklahoma state line, and that was because of the presence of a large multi-specialty group clinic there which provided much of the care for a ten-county region. Had the government made the calculations on a *regional* formula basis, even that one county would have been declared underserved. The small number of active medical practitioners was of special concern because of the unusually large numbers of elderly and disabled persons residing in the most rural areas (Figures 1.A and 1.B).

In 1976 DHEW published a list of *critical* health manpower shortage areas for the nation, taking into account the following published criteria:

... the ratio of resident civilian population of the area to the number of full-time equivalent, non-Federal primary care physicians practicing within the proposed service area (including those practicing in federal-funded neighborhood health centers, local health department clinics, and hospital outpatient departments) must be greater than 4,000:1. Primary care physicians are here defined to include all those physicians (M.D. and D.O.) practicing general or family medicine, internal medicine, pediatrics, and obstetrics and gynecology, and those general surgeons who spend 50 percent or more of their patient care time in primary care practice. (Unless data to the contrary is supplied, general surgeons in nonmetropolitan areas will be assumed to fall in this category ...).

Parts of all of 29 Arkansas counties were listed in this critical designation, as seen in Figure 1.C.

6

**Percent of Total Population 65 Years of Age and Over;
Arkansas by County: 1970**

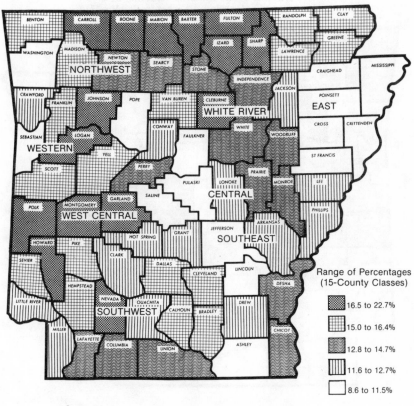

Range of Percentages
(15-County Classes)

16.5 to 22.7%

15.0 to 16.4%

12.8 to 14.7%

11.6 to 12.7%

8.6 to 11.5%

Source:
A Changing Arkansas: Population and Related Data
Prepared by Industrial Research and Extension Center
of the University of Arkansas, Little Rock, p. 19, 1973.

FIGURE 1.A

**Percent of Total Population 16-64 that were
Handicapped or Disabled; Arkansas by County: 1970**

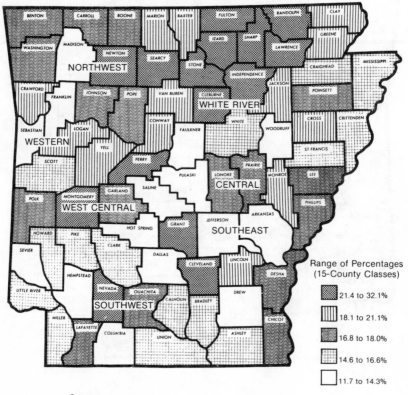

Range of Percentages
(15-County Classes)

- 21.4 to 32.1%
- 18.1 to 21.1%
- 16.8 to 18.0%
- 14.6 to 16.6%
- 11.7 to 14.3%

Source:
A Changing Arkansas: Population and Related Data
Prepared by Industrial Research and Extension Center
of the University of Arkansas, Little Rock, p. 44, 1973.

FIGURE 1.B

8

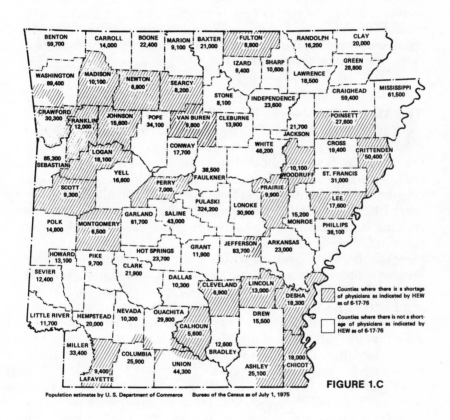

BENTON 59,700	CARROLL 14,000	BOONE 22,400	MARION 9,100	BAXTER 21,000	FULTON 8,800	RANDOLPH 16,200	CLAY 20,000

BENTON
59,700
CARROLL
14,000
BOONE
22,400
MARION
9,100
BAXTER
21,000
FULTON
8,800
RANDOLPH
16,200
CLAY
20,000

IZARD
9,400
SHARP
10,600
GREEN
28,800

WASHINGTON
89,400
MADISON
10,100
NEWTON
6,800
SEARCY
8,200
LAWRENCE
18,500

STONE
8,100
INDEPENDENCE
23,600
CRAIGHEAD
59,400
MISSISSIPPI
61,500

CRAWFORD
30,300
FRANKLIN
12,000
JOHNSON
15,600
POPE
34,100
VAN BUREN
9,800
CLEBURNE
13,900
POINSETT
27,800

21,700
JACKSON

CONWAY
17,700
WHITE
46,200
CROSS
19,400
CRITTENDEN
50,400

85,300
SEBASTIAN
LOGAN
18,100

YELL
16,600
38,500
FAULKNER
10,100
WOODRUFF
ST. FRANCIS
31,000

SCOTT
9,300
PERRY
7,000
PRAIRIE
9,900
LEE
17,600

PULASKI
324,200
LONOKE
30,900

POLK
14,800
MONTGOMERY
6,500
GARLAND
61,700
SALINE
43,000
15,200
MONROE
PHILLIPS
38,100

HOWARD
13,100
PIKE
9,700
HOT SPRINGS
23,700
GRANT
11,900
JEFFERSON
83,700
ARKANSAS
23,000

SEVIER
12,400
CLARK
21,900
DALLAS
10,300
CLEVELAND
6,900
LINCOLN
13,000
DESHA
18,300

LITTLE RIVER
11,700
HEMPSTEAD
20,000
NEVADA
10,300
OUACHITA
29,800
DREW
15,500

MILLER
33,400
CALHOUN
5,600
12,600
BRADLEY

COLUMBIA
25,900
UNION
44,300
ASHLEY
25,100
18,000
CHICOT

9,400
LAFAYETTE

☒ Counties where there is a shortage of physicians as indicated by HEW as of 6-17-76

☐ Counties where there is not a shortage of physicians as indicated by HEW as of 6-17-76

FIGURE 1.C

Population estimates by U. S. Department of Commerce   Bureau of the Census as of July 1, 1975

An analysis of the situation by medical school officials at the time revealed that, indeed, there were major shortages of physicians in many of the towns of the state, and towns which had lost a physician often were left entirely devoid of medical services for months at a time. In other towns those doctors who wanted to retire or reduce their practice could not because nobody could be found to take over their practice. Of most importance, when a new doctor was recruited to a small community there was an enormous risk that he/she would not stay. The problem increasingly came to focus on this last issue, as efforts were begun to recruit new graduates to small town practice. A simple calculation suggested that had the physicians stayed in the communities in which they were recruited, there would have been no deficit at all.

The Major Problem is Rural Medical Retention

The surprising level of turnover in small town physicians was first revealed in a study using annual physician lists compiled by the Arkansas State Medical Board, the licensing agency for the state. Information was compiled on patterns of recruitment and retention within communities of less than 16,000 population* for the years 1962 to 1974. All 635 physicians in the state who were listed as residing in communities of less than 16,000 during the twelve-year period of study are shown in Figure 1.D. Approximately half of these left the practice setting within the twelve-year period at rates inversely proportionate to the size of the community, i.e., the smaller the community, the higher the rate of relocation.

Figure 1.E shows that subset of 304 physicians in the state who left their community within the twelve-year study period, and indicates that the bulk (75%) of attrition took place within the first two years of practice. The table inset shows uniform mobility within the three sizes of communities studied.

Figures 1.F, 1.G and 1.H further summarize the relocation patterns of the 157 physicians who left the communities *within the initial two years of practice.* Those who left after the first two years are included in the "stayed" category in these figures.

The data suggest that about half the small towns in which Arkansas graduates settled did reasonably well in retaining their physicians and satisfying their needs. The other half attracted a doctor for a year or two, lost him, and then began anew the recruitment efforts.

*This included all but 14 communities within the state.

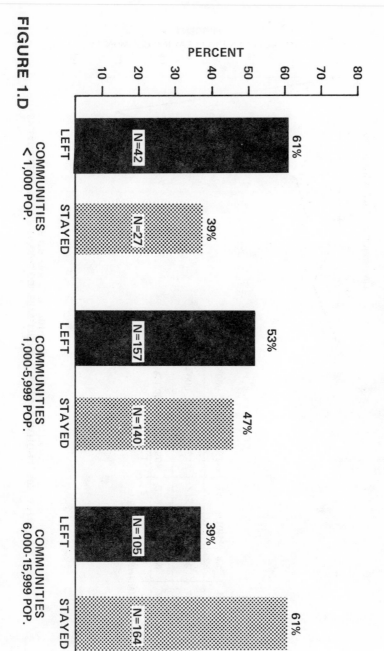

FIGURE 1.D

RETENTION OF PHYSICIANS LOCATING IN ARKANSAS COMMUNITIES OF < 16,000 POPULATION (1962 - 1974)

PERCENT

80 70 60 50 40 30 20 10

61%
LEFT
N=42

39%
STAYED
N=27

COMMUNITIES
< 1,000 POP.

53%
LEFT
N=157

47%
STAYED
N=140

COMMUNITIES
1,000-5,999 POP.

39%
LEFT
N=105

61%
STAYED
N=164

COMMUNITIES
6,000-15,999 POP.

11

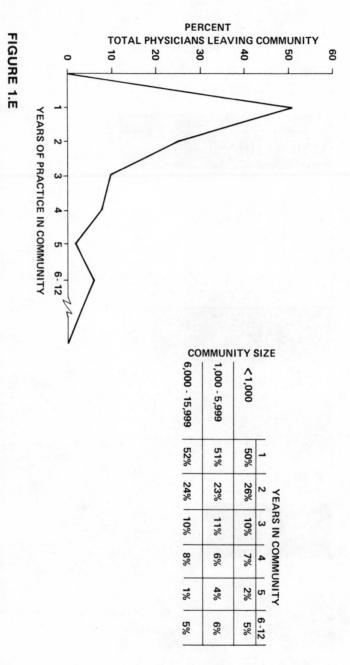

FIGURE 1.E

PHYSICIANS LEAVING ARKANSAS COMMUNITIES < 16,000 POPULATION (1962 - 1974)
BY NUMBER OF YEARS OF PRACTICE IN COMMUNITY

PERCENT
TOTAL PHYSICIANS LEAVING COMMUNITY

YEARS OF PRACTICE IN COMMUNITY

COMMUNITY SIZE	YEARS IN COMMUNITY					
	1	2	3	4	5	6-12
< 1,000	50%	26%	10%	7%	2%	5%
1,000 - 5,999	51%	23%	11%	6%	4%	6%
6,000 - 15,999	52%	24%	10%	8%	1%	5%

12

MOBILITY OF PHYSICIANS IN ARKANSAS DURING
FIRST TWO YEARS OF PRACTICE, 1962 -1974

COMMUNITIES OF LESS THAN 1,000 POPULATION

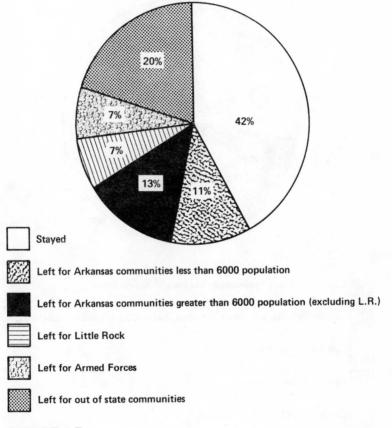

Stayed

Left for Arkansas communities less than 6000 population

Left for Arkansas communities greater than 6000 population (excluding L.R.)

Left for Little Rock

Left for Armed Forces

Left for out of state communities

FIGURE 1.F

MOBILITY OF PHYSICIANS IN ARKANSAS DURING
FIRST TWO YEARS OF PRACTICE, 1962 -1974

COMMUNITIES OF 1,000 -5,999 POPULATION

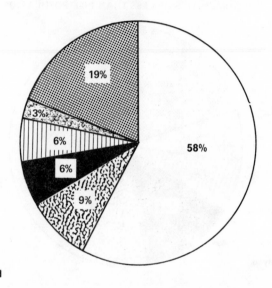

Stayed

Left for Arkansas communities less than 6000 population

Left for Arkansas communities greater than 6000 population (excluding L.R.)

Left for Little Rock

Left for Armed Forces

Left for out of state communities

FIGURE 1.G

14

MOBILITY OF PHYSICIANS IN ARKANSAS DURING FIRST TWO YEARS OF PRACTICE, 1962 -1974

COMMUNITIES OF 6,000 -15,999 POPULATION

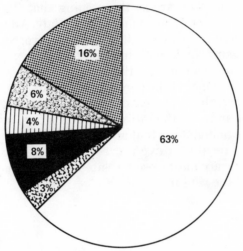

☐ Stayed

▨ Left for Arkansas communities less than 6000 population

■ Left for Arkansas communities greater than 6000 population (excluding L.R.)

▤ Left for Little Rock

▦ Left for Armed Forces

▦ Left for out of state communities

FIGURE 1.H

The High Price of Turnover

The appalling cost to both the physician and to the rural community of this mismatch has not been well described. The young physician and his family moves to the town in good faith, making a long-term commitment. Within weeks or months it becomes apparent that the expectations of the doctor, and sometimes the town, are not to be realized. The agonizing decisions then begin whether to sever the relationship which has been initiated at considerable cost, and to relocate the practice and the family. The lucky doctor makes the break cleanly and moves on to start again; for others the implications of a bad decision are so threatening that the conclusion is rejected, repressed or delayed until it is too late. All too frequently, in that instance, the end result is seen as divorce, alcohol-drug addiction or a similar devastating event.

For the rural community the trauma is almost as great: it is easier in most instances to be perenially without a physician than to find one, go through the process of change in adapting to a new one, lose the doctor and start the entire cycle over again. It is a traumatic process for the human lives that are caught up in the cycle of events, and it is a terribly expensive process for those individuals in the community who are most closely related to the business and financial aspects of the venture.

Chapter 2
Mobility and Other Characteristics of Practicing Physicians

by W. Richard Norton

*... We began to realize very recently that we have been doing
something which ... given the data we know about practice ...
may be destined to failure ... As far as physicians, we have
had limited success ... What can we do, that maintains that
person there? ... what can you do to change the pattern of
isolation, low status and lack of consultation that occurs in
most of the places we are talking about? We feel at the present
time, that without changing those three things, one will not
retain a physician, or any other health professional, beyond
that five-to-seven-year limit when most of the statistics say
they leave. Particularly the young ones.*

> . . . Robert Shannon, M.D.,
> Speaking about the National
> Health Service Corps, 1975.

*Boots — boots — boots —
    movin' up and down again!*

> . . . Rudyard Kipling, "Boots,"
> stanza 1.

The information presented in this chapter and the next stems
from two studies* conducted by the Office of Research, Division of
Rural Medical Development Programs, beginning in the mid-

*W. Richard Norton, John S. Jackson, Diane C. McConnell, Judith A. Jackson and
Thomas A. Bruce, "The Recruitment and Retention of Physicians in Rural Arkansas:
Final Report to the Winthrop Rockefeller Foundation," Part II, 1978.

17

1970's and continuing through the early 1980's. The primary objective of the research was to understand more clearly the dynamics of the physician's selection of a practice location site. The effort involved the collection of relevant data pertaining to the characteristics of Arkansas physicians, both those who chose to practice in rural Arkansas and those who chose to practice in an urban area. The data were collected through two surveys administered to practicing physicians in all counties throughout the state.

Methodology

A questionnaire called the Physician Information Profile (PIP) was designed to provide information on three areas: demographic and background data, training information, and a history of the physician's practice locations, including the dates and the town population size. Although the intent was to administer the questionnaire verbally, it clearly was impossible for the small project staff to interview more than 2,000 practicing physicians in the state and produce the data within a reasonable time span. This difficulty was solved when the University's Cooperative Extension Service indicated an interest in participating in the project. Their system, with staff in each of the 75 Arkansas counties, became a major asset to the careful and timely completion of the study. After a period of training by the project staff, almost all of the interviews were conducted by the County Extension staff members.

Beginning with a list from the Alumni Office of the College of Medicine, and adding other lists from the Department of Health, the Medical Society and the State Medical Board, a state master list of physicians by county was devised; that list contained the names of 2,132 physicians. Completed questionnaires ultimately were returned on 2,108 respondents. Several hundred of these were eliminated in order for the list to contain only practicing physicians (defined as those seeing patients half-time or more). The largest single set eliminated was the group of housestaff physicians still in training; other reasons for elimination were death and retirement. After this reduction, the total number of respondents was 1,709. This was very close to the total number of actively practicing physicians in Arkansas in 1976.

Definition of the word *rural* became an early dilemma. Obviously, the woodlands and pastures of the backcountry would qualify, but such a limited definition was inadequate for a study of medical practice. Similarly, a dusty crossroads community concept was too limited. Neither was the definition satisfactory that has been used in other states, i.e., any town of less than 25,000 population outside a major metropolitan area. Such a definition would have left only nine cities in the state to be classified as nonrural. The population density for Arkansas in 1970 is shown in Figure 2.A.

The final decision was to define any community with less than 16,000 population as rural. Since the term carried a stigma to a number of individuals who lived in towns smaller than 16,000—some viewed it as the equivalent of backward—the terms *metropolitan* and *nonmetropolitan* were used in the questionnaires. This book has returned to the use of the *rural* and *urban* terms, however, because of their easier understanding and ready acceptability.

Population Density; Arkansas by County: 1970

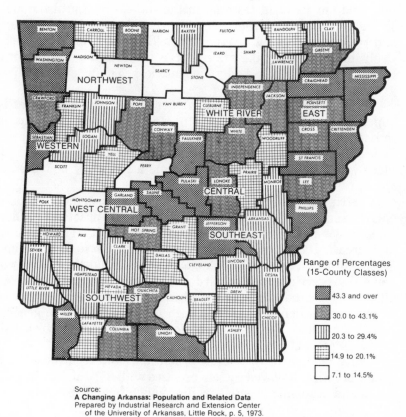

Range of Percentages
(15-County Classes)

- 43.3 and over
- 30.0 to 43.1%
- 20.3 to 29.4%
- 14.9 to 20.1%
- 7.1 to 14.5%

Source:
A Changing Arkansas: Population and Related Data
Prepared by Industrial Research and Extension Center
of the University of Arkansas, Little Rock, p. 5, 1973.

FIGURE 2.A

General Descriptive Information
on Practicing Physicians

Out of the demographic data gathered, a variety of relevant characteristics of Arkansas' active physicians emerged. The primary method for analyzing the data was by statistical frequency and cross-tabulation. The results shown a composite, imaginary physician to be male, middle-aged, and entering his twentieth year of practice. Sixty-nine percent listed Arkansas as their home state. The neighboring states of Tennessee, Missouri, and Texas were given as the state of origin for the next largest groups; only two percent were born outside the United States. Over half (58%) of the total physicians and spouses (56%) in the survey had rural hometowns.

Two of every three physicians practicing in Arkansas received their education in the state's only medical school. Only 36% took internship or resident training in the state. Thus, until the mid-1970's, Arkansas had been a net exporter of physicians for intern and residency training to other states. Since physicians are more likely to practice in the state where they receive postdoctoral training, it is easy to see why the state lost so many of its medical graduates during that time.

Prior to 1976, surgery led the list of specialty disciplines in which residencies were taken (16%); internal medicine was in second place (12%). These were followed at some distance by pediatrics, psychiatry, obstetrics-gynecology and radiology. In seventh place was family practice, at that time a relatively new area of specialty training.

A strikingly different distribution was found on the question of current specialty of practice. Specifically, family practice was indicated by 35% (Table 2.1) of those listing any specialty. This reflected an increasingly common use of the two terms, *family practice* and *general practice*, on an interchangeable basis. That the specialty of general surgery dropped to third place in the list of practice specialties suggests that some of those physicians who took a year or two of surgery residency may have been engaged in a more general (family) practice. The same likely was true of those who took a residency in internal medicine.

Fifty percent of the state's practitioners were involved in a group practice, followed by solo practice with 35%, and by institutional and academic practice trailing much further behind.

Practice Location Patterns

Practice location patterns were defined for those Arkansas physicians in active practice in 1976. On the basis of the individual's chronological history of medical practice, one of six designations was applied to each physician (Figure 2.B). The largest group (41%) of the six had initially settled in an urban area and had never moved; these were labeled Urban. The second largest group (19%) had settled initially in a rural area and never moved (Rural). These two groups together were classified as *nonmovers*. There were four groups who moved from one community to another; intracommunity moves were not included. These latter groups were known as the *movers:* 13% of physicians changed from one urban to another urban community (Urban-to-Urban), 13% moved from a rural community to an urban community (Rural-to-Urban), nine percent (9%) moved from one rural community to another rural site (Rural-to-Rural), and six percent (6%) moved from an urban site to a rural location (Urban-to-Rural).

TABLE 2.1
Type of Specialties Listed By Arkansas Physicians

Specialty Type	Percentage	n
1. Family Practice	35	503
2. Internal Medicine	11	153
3. Surgery - General	8	118
4. Psychiatry	6	83
5. Radiology	5	74
6. Pediatrics	5	69
7. Obstetrics - Gynecology	5	68
8. Ophthalmology	4	58
9. Surgery - Specialized	4	57
10. Orthopedics	4	51
11. General Practice	3	47
12. Anesthesiology	3	46
13. Pathology	3	41
14. Other	3	39
15. Otorhinolaryngology	2	28
16. Dermatology	1	17
	102%*	1452

(n=1452, PIP)
*Percentages do not total 100 because of rounding error.

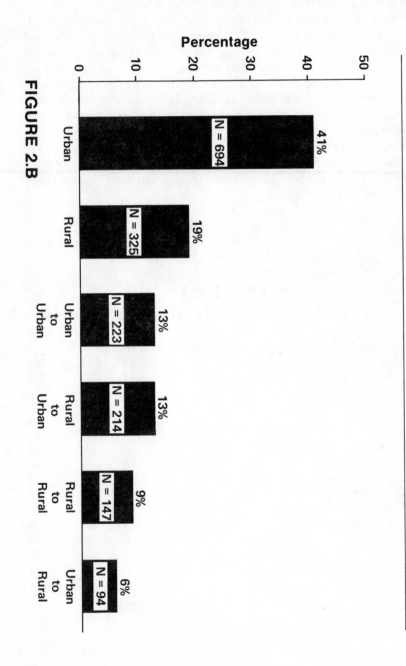

DISTRIBUTION OF ARKANSAS PHYSICIANS ACCORDING TO MOVEMENT PATTERNS

Percentage

FIGURE 2.B

Urban — N = 694 — 41%

Rural — N = 325 — 19%

Urban to Urban — N = 223 — 13%

Rural to Urban — N = 214 — 13%

Rural to Rural — N = 147 — 9%

Urban to Rural — N = 94 — 6%

An amazing 40% of Arkansas physicians thus had moved their practice location from one community to another (Figure 2.C). In addition it can be seen that stability in rural practice settings was half that of urban settings, as measured by the proportion of non-movers in those two categories. Twenty-two percent of physicians had moved only once and 12% had moved twice; 7% had moved their practice three or more times (Figure 2.D). A complete list of the practice location patterns by current specialty is shown in Table 2.2.

Factors Associated with Rural Practice

Now the study turns from general characteristics of the physician population to an analysis of those factors which are associated with practice in a rural area. Although not all are discussed here, Table 2.3 shows the list of factors which were examined.

A male physician was more likely to practice in rural areas than a female physician (42% for males as opposed to 25% for females in the initial practice decision). Having Arkansas as a home state was related to rural practice, although these differences were not large (45% for native Arkansans and 32% for non-Arkansans).

There was a substantial difference in the tendency for rural practice, however, when one compared physicians with a rural hometown with those who had urban hometown backgrounds. Virtually all of the literature indicates that those with rural hometowns are more oriented toward rural practice locations than those from urban hometowns. Arkansas physicians with a rural hometown were more than twice as likely (44% to 19%) to be practicing in a rural area than were those from an urban hometowns (Table 2.4). The same proportion was true of the spouse of a physician. Background is one of the two or three factors most consistently associated with a rural practice.

The training site of a physician also bears some influence on the propensity to practice in rural areas. For example, 38% of those who attended medical school in Arkansas practice in a rural area while only 25% of those who attended an out-of-state medical school do so. Although the site of the postdoctoral training hospital did not correlate closely, taking a residency in family practice or a rotating internship demonstrated a strong statistical relationship with rural practice. This is not surprising since these tend to be the broadest-based postdoctoral training paths in the medical field, providing a solid background for practice in a rural setting. Thus, approximately two-thirds of those who defined their practice specialty as either family practice or general pratice had an end-point location in rural areas (Figure 2.E); an even higher number (three-fourths) of that same group located initially in a rural area (Figure 2.F).

23

Indeed, 72% of all physicians practicing in a rural area are in one of those two specialties (Figure 2.G). It is clear that this is consistently associated with location in a rural area.

Finally, there is an association of solo practice to location in a rural area; this may not necessarily be causal. The relationship may be more that settling in a rural area necessitated a solo practice than that an interest in solo practice led to a rural location.

A tabulation of the end-point practice location for Arkansas physicians in the 1976 study indicated that 33% were in rural areas, while the other 67% were in urban areas (Figure 2.H). It should be noted that about two-thirds of the state's citizens lived outside these urban communities. Thus, one-third of the state's physicians practice in the rural areas where two-thirds of the people live. Although it can be argued reasonably that many of the physicians in urban areas are specialists who serve a much larger population than just that of their own city, this comparison does indicate the crux of the problem.

Movers and Nonmovers in Arkansas Physician Population

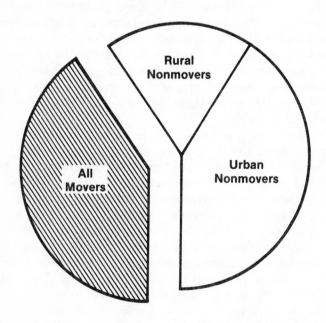

FIGURE 2.C

24

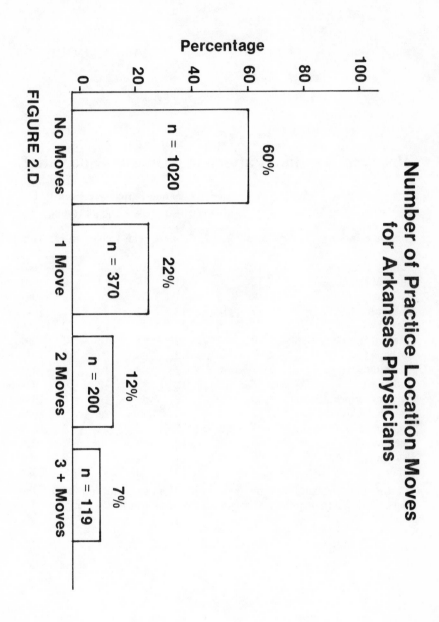

Number of Practice Location Moves
for Arkansas Physicians

FIGURE 2.D

TABLE 2.2
Practice Location Patterns by Current Specialty*

Current Specialty	Practice Location Patterns (percent)						
	Rural	Rural to Rural	Rural to Urban	Urban	Urban to Urban	Urban to Rural	Total
Family Practice	43%	20	10	19	3	5	100%
General Practice	43	19	11	17	4	6	100%
Pathology	12	2	7	51	24	2	98%
Ophthalmology	12	10	12	41	21	7	103%
Surgery - General	12	6	13	44	13	12	100%
Internal Medicine	9	1	9	61	15	4	99%
Orthopedics	8	0	2	63	22	6	101%
Otorhinolaryngology	7	0	4	68	18	0	97%
Radiology	7	7	12	39	12	20	97%
Surgery - Specialized	5	0	9	65	16	5	100%
Anesthesiology	4	2	26	44	22	2	100%
Obstetrics - Gynecology	3	2	7	72	13	3	100%
Dermatology	0	0	12	88	0	0	100%
Psychiatry	0	1	41	34	17	5	99%
Other	8	0	10	49	31	3	101%

*In this table the rows total to 100% (rather than the column totals). Some percentages do not total 100 because of rounding error.

TABLE 2.3
Factors Examined in the
Physician Information Profile

Year of birth
Sex
Hometown of physician
    Population
Hometown of spouse
    Population
Medical school
    Year of graduation
    Institution
    City and State
Internship
    Years
    Type
    Institution
    City and State
Residency
    Years
    Department
    Institution
    City and State
Second Residency
    Years
    Department
    Institution
    City and State
Practice Specialty
Practice Location History
    Community(ies)
    Population of community(ies)
    Dates
Number of communities in which physician works
Proportion of time devoted to practice
Type of practice (solo, etc.)

TABLE 2.4
Practice Location Patterns by Hometown Size

Practice Location Patterns	Hometown Size	
	Rural	Urban
Rural	25%	11%
Urban	32	53
Rural-to-Urban	14	10
Rural-to-Rural	13	3
Urban-to-Rural	6	5
Urban-to-Urban	7	18
	97%*	100%
Total for Physicians Currently Practicing in Rural Areas	44%	19%

*Percentages do not total 100 because of rounding error.

Proportion of Each Specialty in Rural Practice

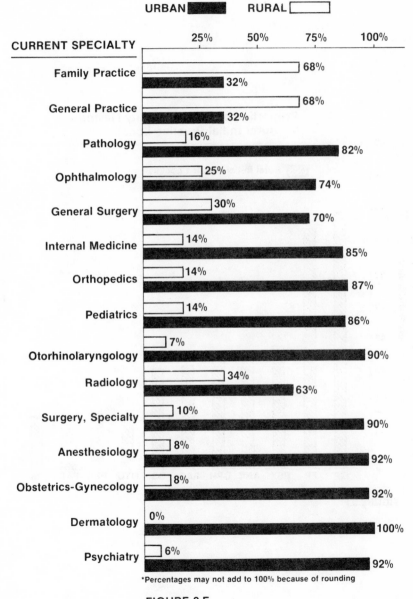

*Percentages may not add to 100% because of rounding

FIGURE 2.E

29

Proportion of Each Specialty Having
Rural Initial Practice Location

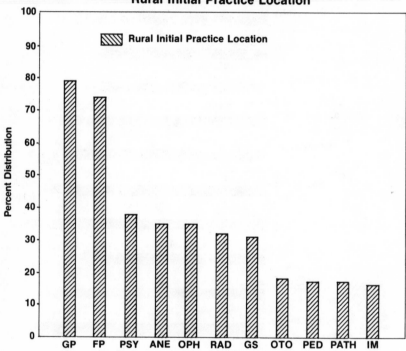

FIGURE 2.F

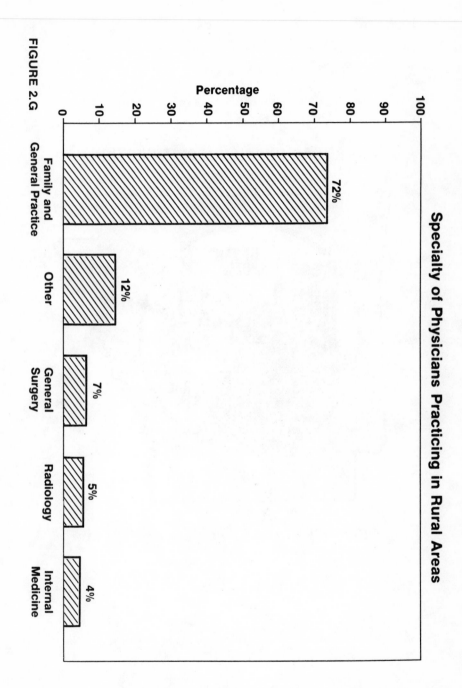

Specialty of Physicians Practicing in Rural Areas

FIGURE 2.G

Percentage

Family and General Practice 72%

Other 12%

General Surgery 7%

Radiology 5%

Internal Medicine 4%

31

ARKANSAS PHYSICIAN DISTRIBUTION

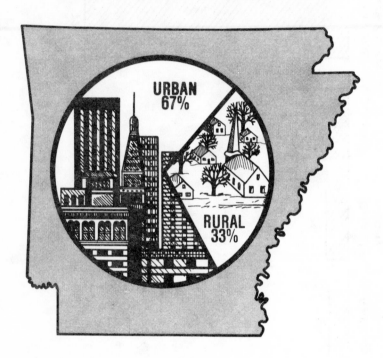

FIGURE 2.H

Chapter 3
Attitudes of Practicing Physicians to Rural Practice

by W. Richard Norton

Physicians occupy an unusual spot in the social structure of rural communities. From an economic standpoint, they are successful entrepreneurs, well-paid business people similar to bankers and lawyers. On the other hand, they are also social servants like policemen or teachers, just as essential to the welfare and functioning of the community but paid for through a fee-for-service mechanism outside of local community control. This anomalous status requires some fairly innovative interpersonal and structural relationships to strike a workable balance.

.... Rosenblatt and Moscovice, 1982

At Rome, you long for the country; when you are in the country, fickle, you extol the absent city to the skies.

.... Horace, *Satires*, Book II, vii

With a large base of data available on state physicians and their sites of practice, it was imperative to understand more clearly why a physician chooses to move into or out of a rural community. Accordingly, a questionnaire was developed (the Physician Change Profile, or PCP)* to explore some of the more pertinent issues. Because of the confidential nature of the material requested in this questionnaire, this second survey was administered by mail. A strong and

---

*W. Richard Norton, John S. Jackson, Diane C. McConnell, Judith A. Jackson and Thomas A. Bruce, "The Recruitment and Retention of Physicians in Rural Arkansas: Final Report to the Winthrop Rockefeller Foundation," Part II, 1978.

positive relationship exists between the state's physicians and the state's only medical school; this was beneficial in obtaining a reasonable response from such a confidential and extensive form. Questionnaires were mailed to the 1,709 physicians who previously had been divided into the six groups of *movers* and *nonmovers*. There were 1,246 returned questionnaires, a response rate of 75%. On analysis, the distribution of respondents from the mail survey was virtually identical to those of the original, more exhaustive interview set (Table 3.1).

This second survey was designed in two parts: the first part dealt with a physician's reasons for choosing a particular initial practice location, rural or urban. The second part probed the factors influencing the physician's decision to move or stay in that location. The survey instrument also included questions dealing with the physicians' perceptions of the adequacy of their training during medical school for various aspects of practicing medicine.

TABLE 3.1
Comparison of Physician Respondents
in the Two Studies

	PIP Physicians		PCP Physicians	
	n	Percentage	n	Percentage
Sex				
Male	1638	96	1194	96
Female	66	4	50	4
Age				
Born before 1940	1359	80	984	80
Born after 1940	330	20	252	20
Medical School				
Arkansas	1176	67	822	67
Other	526	33	397	33
Hometown Size				
Rural (<16,000)	979	58	706	57
Urban(≧16,000)	707	42	530	43
	(n = 1709)		(n = 1246)	

$x^2 = .3565$
p is not significant

The questionnaire borrowed heavily from a 1974 Rand Corporation publication by Heald, Cooper and Coleman, entitled, "Choice of Location of Practice of Medical School Graduates: Analysis of Two Surveys." This seminal report provided a basic understanding of the dynamics of physician location from a national perspective. Several of the questions were drawn conceptually, and sometimes almost verbatim, from the Rand study.

A strong theme dominated both the factors for choosing a rural or urban initial practice location and the factors involved in subsequent decisions to move or stay. This theme centered in the tendency of those who were locating in rural areas to be doing so for personal reasons, while those who were locating in urban areas tended to be doing so for professional reasons. For example, 57% of the doctors who chose a rural practice did so "because it was a non-metropolitan area;" in contrast, the urban nature of the practice was attractive to only 43% of the city dwellers. Table 3.2 shows those factors which were felt to be most important in an initial practice

TABLE 3.2
Rankings of Factors Important in
Initial Practice Location Decision

Factor	1st Place	2nd Place	3rd Place	Total Points
Rural Practice				
Preference for nonmetropolitan living	363	84	27	474
Having been reared in same or similar area	177	94	34	305
High medical need of area	126	110	38	274
Opportunity to join desirable partnership or group practice	87	66	26	179
Climate/geographic features	60	78	37	175
Urban Practice				
Opportunity to join desirable partnership or group practice	273	118	46	437
Ability to limit practice to a specialty	249	110	35	394
Having been reared in same or similar area	228	82	33	343
Preference for metropolitan living	189	68	38	295
Availability of clinical support facilities and personnel	102	102	64	268

location decision, rural or urban. It is clear that "preference for non-metropolitan living" and "having been reared in a similar area" are quite personal reasons for choosing a rural practice site. The "opportunity to join a desirable partnership" and "ability to limit practice," on the other hand, reflect the preponderant professional basis for choosing an urban site.

In addition, for those physicians who elected to continue their initial practice location, the *nonmovers*, all five of the factors most frequently influencing a rural decision are personal (Table 3.3). The only factor in this group not seen in the decisions for an initial rural practice location is "income potential." The list of factors influencing the decision to remain in an urban area reflects the same top three professional reasons as were cited earlier for initiating practice in a city environment.

TABLE 3.3
Ranking of Factors Influencing Decision to Continue Practice in Same Location

Factor	1st Place	2nd Place	3rd Place	Total Points
Rural Group				
Preference for nonmetropolitan living	34	16	10	144
High medical need in area	18	11	12	88
Having been reared in such a community	13	5	8	57
Climate or geographic feature of area	7	14	6	55
Income Potential	8	11	7	53
Urban Group				
Ability to limit practice to a specialty	29	25	18	155
Opportunity to join desirable partnership or group practice	31	13	9	128
Availability of clinical support facilities and personnel	19	21	17	116
Preference for metropolitan living	17	17	11	96
Influence of spouse	16	18	12	96

The *movers*, as indicated in the previous chapter, were separated into Rural-to-Urban, Urban-to-Urban, Rural-to-Rural and Urban-to-Rural groups. Of those four clusters, two were designated as *boundary crossers*, e.g., the Rural-to-Urban and Urban-to-Rural. Almost three-quarters of these boundary crossers left the rural areas for a more urban area. It was an expected trend but the overwhelming proportion was not anticipated by the authors.

The *movers* were asked to write in their own words the major reasons they had moved. Thirty-eight percent of the responses from the Rural-to-Urban group said it was because they wanted to limit their practice to a specialty or had a better offer (Table 3.4). Overwork, better offer, the influence of family and friends, and inadequate income were other reasons given to explain their move.

TABLE 3.4
Written Responses for Practice Location Move

Group	Reason #1	Reason #2
Rural-to-Urban	Ability to specialize (29%)	Had a better offer (9%)
Urban-to-Urban	Had a better offer (21%)	Returned to previously established practice (8%)
Urban-to-Rural	Had a better offer (12%) Overwork (12%)	Influence of family or friends (10%)
Rural-to-Rural	Inadequate facilities (12%)	Inadequate income (10%)

Physicians who had moved were asked to give the degree of influence on their decision for each of the following: a) advantages of the new location; b) disadvantages of the old location; and c) personal reasons. The results can be seen in Table 3.5. In general,

37

TABLE 3.5
Relative Mean Weight of Community/Personal Factors Influencing Move

Factors*	Rural to Urban	Urban to Rural	Rural to Rural	Urban to Urban	Overall
Advantages in the new location	2.77 (n=147)	2.46 (n=50)	2.92 (n=72)	2.66 (n=120)	2.70
Disadvantages in the old location	2.33 (n=144)	1.88 (n=48)	2.60 (n=72)	2.23 (n=117)	2.26
Personal reasons	2.64 (n=143)	2.70 (n=53)	2.57 (n=74)	2.68 (n=118)	2.65

*Responses were 1=no influence,   2=some influence,   3=strong influence   4=very strong influence

physicians in all four groups moved more often because of advantages in the new location, rather than disadvantages in the old location. Personal reasons (reasons other than the location) had a moderately strong influence in the physician's decision to move and may have included a variety of important reasons which were even too confidential to relate in a survey of this type.

In a more in-depth analysis of the community disadvantages which influenced the move, the survey found overwork to be the factor ranked most important for all four groups (Table 3.6). Professional isolation and professional animosity were ranked in the top three by those moving from an urban location (Urban-to-Urban and Urban-to-Rural). Those moving from a rural location (Rural-to-Urban and Rural-to-Rural) also ranked professional isolation, unrealistic public demands and inadequate clinical support in the top three. Overall, there appears to be a great deal of commonality among all four groups and relatively little Urban-to-Rural dichotomy.

Physicians were asked to indicate those factors which were important in their decision to move to another location. This was a forced-choice question where the respondent selected from a list of 26 items. The ranking of the three most important factors in each group is shown in Table 3.7. Both of the groups who moved to a rural location (Rural-to-Rural and Urban-to-Rural) gave a preference for nonmetropolitan living as the most important factor. The Rural-to-Urbans indicated that the ability to limit their practice to a specialty was the most important.

38

TABLE 3.6

Ranking of Community Disadvantages
Which Influenced Move

Factor	1st Place	2nd Place	3rd Place	Total Points
Urban-to-Urban Group				
Overwork	12	4	2	46
Professional Animosity	5	7	3	32
Professional Isolation	7	3	3	30
Urban-to-Rural Group				
Overwork	8	3	1	31
Professional Isolation	1	3	1	10
Professional Animosity	0	3	4	10
Rural-to-Urban Group				
Overwork	38	17	12	160
Professional Isolation	14	31	12	116
Unrealistic Public Demands	13	14	11	78
Rural-to-Rural Group				
Overwork	14	4	6	56
Inadequate clinical support facilities	7	10	4	45
Professional Isolation	6	9	5	41

Most of the physicians said they felt there was nothing the community from which they moved could have done to prevent them from moving. Eighty-four percent of the Rural-to-Urban respondents to this question indicated that nothing could have been done, as did 80% of the Urban-to-Rural and the Urban-to-Urban groups, and as did 70% of the Rural-to-Rural group. Physicians who moved from rural areas mentioned providing adequate hospital and clinical facilities, more support from the community and its leaders, and relief from overwork. The Rural-to-Rural respondents also mentioned specifically the resolution of conflict with partners or hospital administrators.

Other Issues Related to the Decision
to Practice in a Rural Area

Several other matters were studied which might have been pertinent to the rural/urban location decision. On analysis, most of these appear to be ancillary issues and not core areas of major concern. For example, when asked about the influence of their

39

TABLE 3.7
Ranking of Factors Influencing Move

Factor	1st Place	2nd Place	3rd Place	Total Points
Rural-to-Rural Group				
Preference for nonmetropolitan living	15	6	6	63
Income potential	9	7	5	46
Availability of clinical support facilities and personnel	9	2	4	35
Urban-to-Rural Group				
Preference for nonmetropolitan living	13	2	2	45
High medical need in area	3	10	5	34
Climate or geographic feature of area	5	3	4	25
Rural-to-Urban Group				
Ability to limit practice to a specialty	25	12	7	106
Opportunity for regular contact with a specific institution or medical school or center	14	7	7	63
Opportunity to join desirable partnership or group practice	14	7	5	61
Preference for metropolitan living	15	6	4	61
Urban-to-Urban Group				
Preference for metropolitan living	17	7	5	70
Income Potential	12	12	10	70
Climate or geographic feature of area	12	11	12	70

medical school on their practice location choice, most physicians did not view it as a crucial factor. Eighty percent of the respondents initially locating in rural areas and 75% initially locating in urban areas indicated that their medical school was not an important factor in their choice of practice sites. An additional question asked whether their medical training had adequately prepared them for their first practice. A majority of those with both urban (60%) and rural (72%) initial practice locations felt their medical school training had adequately prepared them for their practice needs. Of those who felt they were not adequately prepared, most attributed this inadequacy to the lack of overall medical knowledge (especially in a rural area), to the lack of a preceptorship or other such practical experience, or to a lack of training in the business aspects of practice.

In indicating what their medical school could have done to provide more adequate preparation for practice in a rural area, most respondents suggested preceptorships, AHEC rotation or other actual field experience, more overall experience in practicing medicine broadly and more preparation for business aspects of practice, particularly office management and choosing a practice location.

The physician respondents perceived some generic advantages and disadvantages of an urban or rural setting for a practice. Of the advantages of a rural area, cited by rural respondents, the following were most frequent: preference for rural living per se, better family life, and closer and more rewarding relationships with patients. The disadvantages which they saw in a rural area were those of professional isolation, insufficient facilities, and the inability to practice a specialty of medicine.

The advantages felt to be attributable to a metropolitan area by the urban respondents were the availability of specialty consultation in their practice, the ability to practice one's own specialty, and a preference for urban living. Disadvantages were the personal preference for living in a rural area, too much competition and city congestion.

Summary

Several relevant findings emerged for the analysis of these data. The tendency of physicians to select rural areas for personal reasons and urban areas for professional reasons has again been validated. This was basically true in both the initial practice decision as well as in subsequent relocation. In addition, the preference for rural living for those who chose rural areas, and the preference for urban living for those who chose urban areas is quite strong. Even though this was considered a personal factor, it was consistently high even in the list of reasons for selecting an urban community.

With reference to relocation, there is a tendency, consistent among all four groups of movers, to indicate that the move was because of advantages in the new community, as opposed to disadvantages in the old community. However, when the movers indicated the community disadvantages which influenced the move, all four groups ranked "overwork" first on their list. Moreover, most movers indicated that there was nothing the initial community could have done to hold them.

Chapter 4
Factors Influencing Medical Students and Housestaff Specialty Choice and Planned Practice Location

by Vardelle K. Johnson
and W. Richard Norton

Change is always more troublesome than sitting still. Change is most easily accomplished at the medical school-college interface or in the first two years of medical school. Innovation at this level will never have much effect on the educational program, because the majority of a doctor's education comes after that period of time. Any significant change will have to affect the clinical years of medical school, internship, residency and postgraduate education.

... Eugene A. Stead, Jr., M.D.

The residency is a period of unbelievable professional growth and development, and with good fortune, may even be accompanied by comparable logarithmic personal enlargement. The resident should make a knowing and informed commitment to be a physician: to take care of patients with compassion, justice, honor, dignity, scholarship and devotion.

... Solomon Papper, M.D.,
Doing Right, 1983.

The students and housestaff (interns, residents and fellows) of the College of Medicine, University of Arkansas for Medical Sciences, were surveyed on two occasions to elicit their perceptions of factors which were important in the selection of a specialty and in

the consideration of a future practice location. The first questionnaire was mailed in March, 1977, to all 483 students and 288
members of the housestaff; the second was mailed in March, 1980,
but only to the 345 members of the housestaff. Because of the basic
differences in the status of a medical student and a resident physician, these two groups were separated for purposes of analysis.

Comparison of Medical Student and Housestaff Attitudes (1977 Survey)

Responses were received from 397 students, a response rate of
82%. The majority (84%) of the students were male and ranged in age
from 22 to 38, with the mean age being 26 years. Fifty-one percent
were married. Slightly over half (54%) were from urban hometowns, and 60% of the spouses were from urban hometowns. The
majority (88%) of the students and their spouses (66%) were Arkansas natives.

Of the 288 housestaff surveyed, 193 returned questionnaires,
yielding a response rate of 67%. A majority (91%) again were male,
and ages ranged from 24 to 43, with a mean age of 30 years. Seventy-
nine percent were married. Most of the housestaff (72%) and their
spouses (63%) were from Arkansas. Over half (58%) were from
urban hometowns as were the spouses (59%).

Many similarities were seen between the student and housestaff surveys; a few potentially important differences were
observed. The majority of both groups were undecided about a
specific practice location. As expected, the percentage for housestaff who were undecided was smaller (65%) than for students (87%).
Housestaff members were nearer the completion of their training
and thus the selection of a future practice location was more immi-
nent. But while most (67%) of the housestaff preferred an urban
practice, the students were about equally divided between urban
(41%) and rural (38%) practice preference (Table 4.1). Interest in the
potential of a rural practice site was reasonably constant through
all four years of medical education (Figure 4.A).

The literature indicates a strong influence of hometown on
practice location. Fifty-five percent of the students and 33% of the
housestaff in the survey who were from rural hometowns preferred
a future rural practice, in contrast to the interest in a rural practice
of only 24% of students and 12% of housestaff from urban hometowns. It was also evident in both groups that those with spouses
from rural hometowns (54% in students, 30% in housestaff) were
more likely to be planning rural practice than those with spouses
from urban hometowns (36% in students, 12% in housestaff). There
was a proclivity among respondents with spouses who were reared

44

TABLE 4.1
Medical Student Preference of Practice Location Size

Rural	n	Percentage
Less than 1,000	2	1
1,000 - 2,499	13	3
2,500 - 5,999	51	13
6,000 - 9,999	33	8
10,000 - 15,999	51	13
Total	150	38

Urban	n	Percentage
16,000 - 24,999	31	8
25,000 - 49,999	49	12
50,000 - 99,999	28	7
100,000 - 499,999	49	12
500,000 - 999,999	4	1
1,000,000 and over	3	1
Total	164	41
Undecided	81	20

Medical Student Year in Training by Preferred Practice Location Size

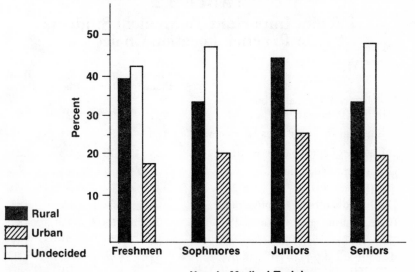

FIGURE 4.A

45

in Arkansas to prefer rural practice as opposed to those reared outside the state. These findings replicate those on practicing Arkansas physicians presented in Chapter 2 of this book.

A great deal of consideration was being given by the survey respondents to the interests of their spouses in the selection of a future practice location. An overwhelming majority (93%) of both students and housestaff indicated that spouse considerations would play an influential role in their consideration of a practice location. The most frequently cited specific considerations in both groups were the spouse's "career opportunities," "social/cultural opportunities," and "general preference for either rural or urban location."

As is generally known, group practice was the organizational type of practice preferred by both students and housestaff. Only a small portion of each group was planning to practice solo, irrespective of the potential interest in a rural or urban practice site.

The medical students listed several factors as most important in their future decision to choose a practice site (Table 4.2). The personal preference for rural or urban living was indicated as the single most important factor. Next in order were "climate and geographic preferences," "spouse influence" and "opportunity for group practice." Only the latter issue is a professional reason for

TABLE 4.2
Factors Important To Medical Students
In Practice Location Choice*

Factor	1st Place	2nd Place	3rd Place	Total Points
Preference for rural/urban living (Personal)	261	78	21	360
Climate/geographic area (Personal)	123	120	61	304
Influence of spouse (Personal)	123	78	23	224
Group practice option (Professional)	114	52	30	196
High medical need (Professional)	105	54	27	186
Clinical support (Professional)	78	58	21	157
Cultural and social life (Personal)	54	52	31	137
Schools for children (Personal)	24	70	26	120

*Rating code: 1st place-3 points, 2nd place-2 points, 3rd place-1 point.

46

selecting a rural/urban site for practice, and the medical students seemed to rank it a weaker factor than the other more personal concerns which they or their spouse felt. These results are comparable to the housestaff surveys (see below), but the issues of professional concern seem to weigh more heavily as the physicians progress in training.

Specialty choice is another major factor which is known to be a powerful predictor in the direction of rural practice. The study revealed that one of the primary care specialties—family practice, internal medicine, or pediatrics—was preferred by 60% of the students and 43% of the housestaff. Since family practice is the specialty with an enormous lead over any other specialty in terms of its correlation with rural practice, a special analysis was made of this discipline. Irrespective of the year in training, family practice was the most popular specialty among medical students (Table 4.3). It is interesting to note, however, the difference in percentages for each class; the proportion of those preferring family practice drops from 52% in the freshman class to 29% in the senior class, a substantial fall!

The housestaff were about equally divided with regard to faculty influence on their specialty choice (51% seemed to think that faculty were important in the decision). This influence, when

TABLE 4.3
Medical Student Year in Training
by Specialty Choice

	Year in Medical Training			
Specialty	Freshman %	Sophomore %	Junior %	Senior %
Family Practice	52	32	29	29
Internal Medicine	9	20	12	21
Pediatrics	8	14	6	9
Surgery	8	4	9	5
General Practice	1	8	12	3
Obstetrics-Gynecology	3	5	6	6
Psychiatry	0	2	5	5
Radiology	2	2	4	2
Pathology	0	1	3	2
Anesthesiology	1	0	0	5
Other	15	10	13	14
Total	99%*	98%*	99%*	101%*

*Do not equal 100 due to rounding

present, seemed to emanate from a specific individual faculty member. Faculty influence was judged somewhat higher on specialty choice than on practice location selection, where both students and housestaff agreed that faculty played a relatively small role.

The relationship between hometown and specialty choice was examined, and results showed that medical students from rural hometowns (45%) were much more likely than students from urban hometowns (28%) to choose family practice. In addition, male students were more likely than female students to choose family practice. The marital status was found to be important only in the tendency for more single than married students to select surgery as a specialty discipline. In examining residents on these issues, no significant differences were found when hometown, sex, and marital status were cross-tabulated with specialty choice.

Cross-tabulation also was used to analyze the dependent variables of practice location site (rural/urban) and the specialty choice (Table 4.4). Of all medical students planning rural practice, almost six out of ten were interested in family practice in comparison to only two of ten for those who were planning to practice in an urban area. An additional 14% of those planning a rural practice chose·

TABLE 4.4
Medical Student Practice Location Size Preference by Specialty

Specialty	Practice Location Size		
	Rural %	Urban %	Undecided %
Family Practice	57	20	29
Internal Medicine	11	18	18
Pediatrics	8	9	11
Surgery	3	10	6
General Practice	14	2	1
Obstetrics-Gynecology	1	9	4
Psychiatry	1	3	7
Radiology	1	5	1
Pathology	1	2	3
Anesthesiology	0	3	1
Other	5	18	19
Total	102%*	99%*	100%

*Do not equal 100 due to rounding

general practice (an abbreviated residency training) in comparison to only 2% of those planning an urban location. Of the housestaff planning rural practice, the largest number were in family practice (44%), followed by general practice (15%). These two disciplines accounted for over half of those residents planning a rural location.

The conclusions of the 1977 study were:

1) A decision about where to practice was not made until late in the residency years, although both students and housestaff did have very definite preferences for the size of the community in which they planned to practice. The students were about equally divided between a preference for rural and urban practice, but the majority of the housestaff were planning urban practice.

2) Students and housestaff who were in family practice or general practice were more likely to be planning rural practice than those in other specialties.

3) There was a favorable attitude by housestaff toward rural practice, even though most had urban practice plans.

4) The influence of hometown was found to be substantial for both students and housestaff, with a higher proportion of those from rural hometowns planning rural practice than those from urban hometowns. In addition, the influence of the spouse's hometown was also found to be great, with respondents whose spouses were from rural hometowns being more likely to be planning rural practice than those with spouses from urban hometowns.

5) Group practice was planned by the majority of both students and housestaff.

6) Factors considered to be most important in the selection of a practice location were preference for rural or urban living, climate and geographic preference, opportunity for group practice and spouse influence.

Serial Housestaff Attitudinal Surveys (1977 and 1980)

The same questionnaire that was administered in 1977 was used in a follow-up study in 1980. All 345 housestaff in 1980 received the questionnaire, and the response rate (63%) was analogous to that of the earlier survey. The results, shown in Table 4.5, were virtually unchanged from those of the 1977 study with the notable exception of a shift in the ranking of factors important in selecting a practice location. The decision about a practice location still was being made late in training. Group practice still was the preferred type of practice. Although favorable attitudes existed toward practicing and living in rural areas, most housestaff nevertheless were planning an

TABLE 4.5
Comparison of 1977 and 1980 Housestaff

	1977	1980
Response rate	67%	63%
Sex	91% Male	84% Male
Age	24-43 yrs., Mean = 30	23-48 yrs., Mean = 30
Marital status	79% Married	75% Married
Hometown	58% Urban	55% Urban
Homestate	72% Arkansas	67% Arkansas
Spouse hometown	59% Urban	60% Urban
Spouse homestate	63% Arkansas	52% Arkansas
Group practice interest	72% Yes	70% Yes
Specific practice location already made	65% No	70% No
If yes, to specific practice location	73% Urban	77% Urban
Attitude toward rural practice	52% Favorable	54% Favorable
Tending toward urban practice	67%	64%
Tending toward rural practice	20%	20%
Home size	67% Rural	72% Rural
Spouse hometown size	63% Rural	61% Rural
Rural practice preference by specialty	44% Family Practice 14% General Practice 10% Pediatrics	51% Family Practice 16% Internal Medicine 12% General Practice
Important factors - location	Preference for rural/ urban living Group practice option Climate/geographic area Spouse	Spouse Preference for rural/ urban living Climate/geographic area Group practice option
Spouse influence - practice location	93% Yes	94% Yes
Reasons for spouse influence	Consideration of wants/ needs Career opportunity Social/cultural opportunities	Career opportunity Consideration of wants/ needs Family considerations

urban practice (Figure 4.B). The exceptions were those in family practice who were not so specialized that they required a large patient population area to support their practice. Those who grew up in small towns and whose spouses grew up in small towns were much more likely to go back to rural areas to practice.

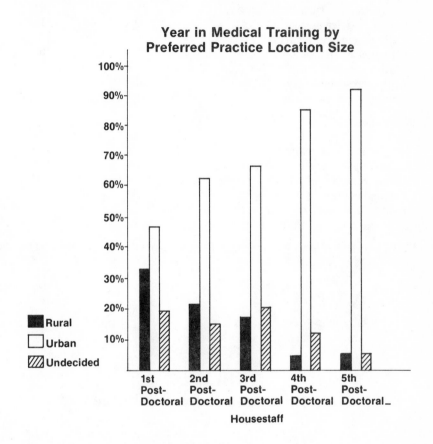

FIGURE 4.B

In the survey of factors important in the practice location choice, spouse influence was at the bottom of the top three concerns in 1977, but was at the top of the list in 1980 (Table 4.6). The perceived reasons for spouse preferences in the site of practice were much like those in the earlier study (Table 4.7). The physicians' preference for living in a rural or urban area still was important, as were climate and geographic preferences and the opportunity for group practice.

51

TABLE 4.6
Factors Important in Practice Location Choice*

1977 Housestaff	1st Place	2nd Place	3rd Place	Total Points
Preference for rural/urban living	105	26	10	141
Group practice option	72	28	12	112
Climate/geographic area	69	18	20	107
Influence of spouse	57	36	10	103
Clinical support	30	28	16	74
Ability to specialize	54	12	8	74
Cultural and social life	9	42	15	66
1980 Housestaff				
Influence of spouse	117	42	10	169
Preference for rural/urban living	123	32	13	168
Climate/geographic area	57	54	32	143
Group practice option	63	34	12	109
Clinical support	24	30	24	78
Ability to specialize	45	20	10	75
Cultural and social life	27	26	22	75

*Rating code: 1st place - 3 points, 2nd place - 2 points, 3rd place - 1 point.

TABLE 4.7
Factors Important in Spouse Influence*

1977 Housestaff	1st Place	2nd Place	3rd Place	Total Points
Consideration of wants/needs	129	14	2	145
Career opportunity	63	8	0	71
Cultural/social life	42	18	2	62
Close to family	33	16	0	49
1980 Housestaff				
Career opportunity	135	8	0	143
Consideration of wants/needs	105	14	0	119
Family considerations	27	26	0	53
Close to family	30	8	1	39

*Rating code: 1st place - 3 points, 2nd place - 2 points, 3rd place - 1 point.

Tracking Analysis: Attitudinal Changes

Thirty-eight of the senior medical students in 1977 were still present at the University of Arkansas Medical Center in 1980 and were finishing residency programs in the primary care specialties (family practice, pediatrics, internal medicine). Because most of those finishing residency programs in these disciplines were in the process of making decisions about their future practice locations, a comparison was made between the responses they gave to the 1980 survey and those given in 1977.

Thirty-four of the 38 remaining at the University Hospital responded to the 1980 survey; Table 4.8 summarizes the comparison of their responses with those given in the earlier study. Group practice

TABLE 4.8

Comparison of Responses of Third-Year Residents with Previous responses as Senior Medical Students

	Seniors	Third-Year Residents
Total respondents	34	34
Sex	85% Male	85% Male
Marital status	68% Married	79% Married
Hometown	53% Rural	53% Rural
Homestate	94% Arkansas	94% Arkansas
Spouse hometown	62% Urban	48% Urban
Group practice	79% Yes	68% Yes
Practice location preference	41% Urban 38% Rural	61% Urban 15% Rural
Rural practice location preference	38%	15%
Hometown size	77% Rural	100% Rural
Spouse hometown size	56% Rural	100% Rural
Attitude toward rural practice	76% Favorable	47% Favorable
Rural practice preference by specialty	39% Family Practice 23% Internal Medicine 23% Pediatrics	40% Family Practice 20% Internal Medicine 20% Pediatrics
Important factors - practice location	Spouse Preference for rural/ urban living	Preference for rural/ urban living Spouse
Reasons for spouse influence	Consideration of wants/ needs Career opportunity	Career opportunity Consideration of wants/ needs

still was preferred by the majority although the percentage was less than in 1977. More were planning urban locations (61%) than in 1977 (41%). This is not too surprising a change since results of previous studies have shown that the likelihood of urban practice increases with further postgraduate training. The percentage of those who were favorable toward rural practice (46%) dropped considerably from those favorable in 1977 (76%). This probably reflects the increased focus on professional support systems, and therefore of the expanded interest in urban practice. Only 15% in comparison to an earlier 38% were actually planning rural practice in 1980. The relationship between rural practice preference and hometown size (including spouse's hometown) still was apparent. All (100%) of those planning a rural practice were from rural hometowns, as were their spouses. Those planning rural practice were primarily in family practice, followed by internal medicine and pediatrics. The reasons for choosing a practice location had not changed, with preference for a rural or urban area and spouse being the two most important concerns.

Overall, the responses given in 1977 as senior medical students were generally reflective of how they felt three years later as senior resident physicians. The only significant change had been the increased interest in an urban practice after three years of additional training at the housestaff level.

Conclusions from the Study

Rural communities who are seeking young, new physicians would do well to focus on those who have rural backgrounds, are in family practice residencies or who are interested in only one year of postdoctoral (internship) training. Group practice opportunities are a strong attraction even to rural practice and the recruitment of the spouse, especially in terms of career opportunities, is probably just as important as the efforts made to recruit the physician.

Chapter 5
Factors Influencing
Recruitment and Retention
in Two Types of Rural Communities

by Diane C. McConnell, James M. Kohls and
W. Richard Norton

*. . . major changes in the distribution of physician services
will not come about until policies that are designed to re-
distribute medical services recognize that a major locus of
the problem is in general differences between communities
and not solely in the attitudes, motives, values, and other
personal characteristics of individual physicians.*

. . . William A. Rushing, 1975

The impetus for the community studies came from several
months experience in working with Arkansas towns needing physicians; it was obvious after a time that some towns had been quite
successful in recruiting and retaining doctors, while other apparently similar towns had difficulty recruiting and retaining over the
years. The question which emerged from this experience was what
made one community so much more attractive than another to
physicians who wanted a small town practice.

First Community Study
A preliminary study of 29 Arkansas communities was undertaken. The communities ranged in population from 1,653 to 11,750.
Fourteen of these communities were chosen because of their high
physician-to-population ratio and their successful retention of
physicians over the past 20 years. Fifteen other communities were
chosen because they had low physician-to-population ratios and had

not had a successful record of retaining physicians during that time.

To insure that the communities chosen did indeed represent the extremes, a panel of experts on community medical affairs in Arkansas was consulted. The purpose was to determine if any of the communities were selected inappropriately, such as a community being low in supply and retention of physicians because of its proximity to a larger city where abundant medical care was available. Deletions were made from the initial list when three of the four panel members agreed.

Measurements of community characteristics were gathered from census data and from publications of several state agencies. The mean values of these data characteristics for each group of communities were compared, and ten of the twenty variables measured were found to differ significantly (Table 5.1). Those fifteen com-

TABLE 5.1

Community Variables	Group 1 Mean	Group 2 Mean	Significance of t Values (two-tailed test)
Demographic			
Population	5335	3524	.104
Median Age	37.3	33.1	.129
% Under Age 5	7.1	8.1	.026*
% Over Age 65	19.3	16.9	.258
% County Urban	29.2	36.5	.358
Miles to Urban Center	51.7	42.7	.329
% White	95.0	74.5	.008*
Economic-Industrial			
Med. Family Income	$6337	$5262	.003*
Unemployment Rate	8.1	8.2	.968
Bank Deposits (in mil.)	$29.79	$11.29	.009*
Retail Sales (in mil.)	$81.42	$50.17	.224
% Inc. in Retail Sales	22.1	14.4	.009*
% Professionals	11.7	10.3	.309
% White Collar	37.4	31.8	.018*
% Farm Labor	2.8	6.3	.043*
% Manufacturing	25.4	27.9	.519
Educational			
Med. Yrs. Educ.	10.9	9.4	.001*
Per Pupil Expen. for Educ.	$800	$866	.266
Medical			
Mi.to Nearest Hospital	2.6	10.0	.029*
# Hospital Beds Per 1,000	13.8	5.1	.010*

*Indicates significance at the .05 level.

56

munities which were less able to attract and retain physicians were more likely to fall in the eastern or southern parts of the state, the Delta farming area or the heavily forested Coastal Plains area (Figure 5.A). The mean population for the unsuccessful communities was 3,523, compared with a mean population of 5,335 for the successful communities, and 40% of the unsuccessful communities had hospitals, compared to 86% of the successful communities. The residents of the communities which had difficulty in attracting and retaining physicians had significantly fewer years of education, a higher percentage were under five years of age, and a higher percentage were non-white. The economic prosperity of the unsuccessful communities also differed—residents had a lower median income, there were fewer white collar workers and more people were engaged in farm labor. Bank deposits in the unsuccessful communities were significantly less, and there was a smaller increase in retail sales over the past ten years.

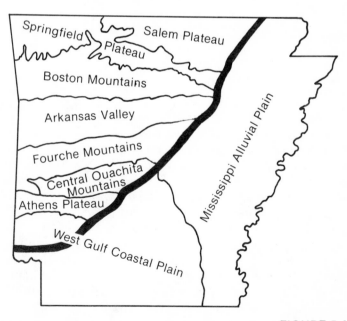

FIGURE 5.A

The relationship between the individual factors of significance was studied to determine which variables discriminated between the successful and the unsuccessful community groups. The results are shown in Table 5.2. Multivariate discriminate analysis found four variables to be most powerful in discriminating between Group 1 and Group 2. The percentage of whites in the community population was shown to be the most important factor, followed by median years of education, proximity to the nearest hospital and the percentage of white collar workers in the labor force.

TABLE 5.2
Most Powerful Community Variables as Determined by Discriminant Analysis

Variable	Wilks' Lambda	Standarized Discriminant Function Coefficients	Significance
% White	.66647	0.57281	0.001
Median Years Education	.54178	0.32793	0.000
Km. to Hospital	.49916	−0.33248	0.001
% White Collar	.47087	0.28171	0.001

Eighty-six percent of the cases were correctly classified by these four variables. Table 5.3 gives the discriminant function score for each community. Community 7 and Community 10, assigned to the Group 1 successful communities, were shown to resemble more closely those in Group 2 when the four variables were considered. Communities 15 and 26, assigned to the Group 2 unsuccessful communities, were shown on the basis of the four discriminating variables to be more like those in Group 1.

An interesting comparison can be made by contrasting the values of these four misclassified communities with their group means for the four variables identified by the discriminant analysis in Table 5.4. Community 7 appeared to differ most with regard to percentage of whites in the population, while Community 10 appeared to differ most in its distance from the nearest hospital.

What that means is that forces are at play in communities which are highly successful at recruiting and retaining physicians which blunt the inherent problems or limitations in the community environment.

Community 15 and Community 26 were misclassified according to the discriminant analysis into Group 2 unsuccessful communities. Such results indicate the presence of personal and other factors at risk even in those communities in which there are synergistic influences of community racial composition, economic and educational prosperity, and occupational structure.

TABLE 5.3
Community Discriminant Scores
(using the four most powerful community variables)

Case	Community Group	Discriminant Function Scores
Community 1	Successful	1.484
Community 2	Successful	1.374
Community 3	Successful	1.761
Community 4	Successful	0.307
Community 5	Successful	1.028
Community 6	Successful	0.257
*Community 7	Successful	−0.251
Community 8	Successful	0.478
Community 9	Successful	0.279
*Community 10	Successful	−0.431
Community 11	Successful	0.449
Community 12	Successful	0.631
Community 13	Successful	1.532
Community 14	Successful	1.460
*Community 15	Unsuccessful	0.291
Community 16	Unsuccessful	−0.194
Community 17	Unsuccessful	−0.188
Community 18	Unsuccessful	−0.817
Community 19	Unsuccessful	−0.525
Community 20	Unsuccessful	−2.166
Community 21	Unsuccessful	−0.991
Community 22	Unsuccessful	−1.594
Community 23	Unsuccessful	−1.448
Community 24	Unsuccessful	−0.578
Community 25	Unsuccessful	−0.637
*Community 26	Unsuccessful	0.284
Community 27	Unsuccessful	−0.563
Community 28	Unsuccessful	−1.187
Community 29	Unsuccessful	−0.047

*Community which does not fit in the group mean

In spite of these exceptions, this preliminary study provided overall support for our hypothesis that the ability of a community to attract physicians was closely related, in general, to the viability* of that community. The data, however, were drawn from secondary sources and several of the measurements had been taken from countywide assessments because the information on the smaller towns themselves was not available. A more in-depth examination of community "wellness" was apparently needed.

TABLE 5.4
Comparison of "Misclassified" Communities

Variables	Group 1 Mean	Successful Communities Misclassified by Discriminant Analysis	
		Community 7	Community 10
% White	95.0	66.2	99.9
Years Education	10.9	10.1	10.3
Miles to Hospital	2.6	0.0	25.0
% White Collar	37.4	34.7	29.3

Variables	Group 2 Mean	Unsuccessful Communities Misclassified by Discriminant Analysis	
		Community 15	Community 26
% White	74.5	71.5	75.3
Years Education	9.4	11.3	11.0
Miles to Hospital	10.0	0.0	0.0
% White Collar	31.8	37.1	36.3

Second Community Study

The opportunity to develop an expanded community study was made possible with a special supplement to College of Medicine funds by the Economics, Statistics and Cooperative Service, Economic Development Division, United States Department of Agriculture. Since resources did not permit an in-depth study of all 29 communities, it was decided to concentrate on two representative towns in some depth. It was intended to test the hypothesis that a community's ability to attract and retain physicians is related to its overall viability. More specifically, the hypothesis was that a community successful in meeting its need for physicians would 1) rate high in its ability to solve other community problems, 2) have a high

*The term community viability is attributed to Roland Warren, who defines it as a community's ability to confront problems and take necessary action. See "Toward a Non-Utopial Normative Model of the Community," American Sociological Review, 35:219-27, 1970.

degree of "communityness" (defined as the residents' identification with their community), and 3) have a wide distribution of decision-making power.

In order to control as many socio-economic variables as possible, communities with similar characteristics were chosen. Although there were certain variations between the two communities chosen, there were a great number of similarities. Both communities are in the same geographic region of the state; both are county seats. They were almost identical in population, and both had accredited hospitals. The difference, however, in the number of physicians in the two communities was distinct: Community *Alpha* had four physicians while Community *Beta* had eight.

An analysis was carried out by means of a questionnaire sent to residents randomly selected from the telephone directories of each town. After a period of pre-testing to validate the instrument, the final questionnaire was mailed in July, 1980, to 906 residents of Alpha and 893 residents of Beta. One-half the cover letters requested that the questionnaire be completed by an adult female, if one were present, and one-half requested that an adult male complete the questionnaire.

Interviews were conducted with the director of the Chamber of Commerce and with the hospital administrators of both communities. Various measurements of community characteristics were gathered from census data and from publications of several state agencies.

Community Problem Solving. Three questions on the questionnaire sent to residents represented an assessment of each community's ability to solve local problems. First, residents were asked to rate their community in its ability to identify and solve local problems. Second, residents were asked to list up to five successful community efforts over the past three years. Third, residents were asked if they could recall more *successes* or more *failures* over the past three years in community efforts to solve local problems.

Residents of Beta consistently rated their community higher on all measurements of community problem-solving ability. Table 5.5 compares the mean value of Alpha and Beta for the three variables measuring community problem-solving ability and shows that all three differed significantly. This disparity held true in spite of the differences in the respondent's income, race, sex and length of residence in the town.

Identification with Community. In order to assess the residents' identification with their community, respondents were asked where they most often purchased various items or services and where they usually went for entertainment. Residents also were asked to write in the town or community in which they worked, if they worked outside the home. In addition, residents' membership in local clubs and organizations and their voting participation was used as a measure of community ties.

TABLE 5.5
Mean Values for Community Problem Solving*

	Mean for Community Alpha	Mean for Community Beta	Significance of T-Value
Ranking of Problem-Solving Ability (Range = 1 to 5)	3.2	4.3	.000
Number of Successful Efforts Listed (Range = 0 to 8)	3.1	3.8	.003
More Community Successes or Failures? (Range = 1 to 3)	2.3	2.7	.000

*Scores ranged from Very Poor (1) to Very Active (5)

The percentages of respondents who obtained goods and services in their own community is shown in Table 5.6 along with the mean number of items which were checked for each town. There was little difference between the two communities with regard to their pattern of obtaining goods and services. Work location, Table 5.7, showed only a slight difference. Beta residents were somewhat more likely (54%) to belong to local clubs or organizations than Alpha residents (50%) and they belonged to a greater number. They also were more likely to vote in local, state and national elections than were residents of Alpha (Table 5.8).

Broad Distribution of Decision-Making Power. Respondents were asked to list the community leaders they would expect to be involved in a community drive or fund raising event and to give the profession of those individuals. More than one concept was being addressed: Could residents clearly identify the leadership of their community, was the leadership of the community in the hands of a few or many and did community leadership reside in one specific sector of the community, such as the business community, churches or schools?

The results were quite similar in identifying leaders for both communities, although Beta residents identified more leaders than Alpha (Table 5.9).

TABLE 5.6
Shopping Patterns

	Percentage of Alpha Residents Who Obtained Goods Or Services in Alpha	Percentage of Beta Residents Who Obtained Goods Or Services in Beta
Groceries	98.1%	97.2%
Clothing, Shoes	64.2	70.4
Furniture	71.4	70.4
Appliances	84.9	77.2
Hardware	91.5	94.5
Dental Work	91.7	84.4
Pharmacy	98.1	93.6
Doctor	76.1	71.9
Hospital	71.1	66.4
Automobiles	77.0	66.4
Auto Repair	91.5	87.8
Gas	97.4	94.9
Bank	97.4	96.4
Insurance	87.7	88.4
Restaurant	48.6	76.7
Entertainment	35.6	56.1
Mean Number of Items	12.2	11.6

TABLE 5.7
Work Location

	Percentage of Alpha Residents Employed in Alpha	Percentage of Beta Residents Employed in Beta
Husband	84%	87%
Wife	94	85
Other Family Member (A)	80	91
Other Family Member (B)	67	100

TABLE 5.8
Voting Patterns

	% Alpha Residents Who Voted in Elections	% Beta Residents Who Voted in Elections
Local Elections	86%	91%
State Elections	88	92
National Elections	86	91

TABLE 5.9
Identification of Leadership

	Alpha	Beta
Identified at least one community leader	62%	69%
Identified at least two community leaders	50	60
Identified at least three community leaders	45	47
Identified at least four community leaders	32	38

The distribution of leadership in particular was not noticeably different (Table 5.10). Eighty-three different individuals were listed as community leaders by respondents of both communities. The only individual to be named by more than one-tenth of the respondents was the mayor in each of the respective communities.

TABLE 5.10
Profession of Community Leaders
Identified Most Frequently By Respondents

Alpha		Beta	
Mayor	16%	Mayor	22%
Banker	5	Banker #1	8
Merchant #1	5	Banker #2	6
Businessman	5	County Judge	6
Merchant #2	4	School Superintendent	6
Minister	4	Banker #3	5
State Representative	4	Retired Merchant	4
Attorney	4	Merchant	4

Characteristics of Respondents. Table 5.11 compares the residents of the two communities who responded to our questionnaire. The Alpha respondents were slightly older, had somewhat less education, had lived in their community longer, and had less household income than the residents of Beta. The percentage of responses from blacks was higher in Alpha than in Beta, as was the percentage of responses from men. Beta had a higher percentage of respondents who were in professional and technical positions than Alpha.

TABLE 5.11
Comparison of Respondents

	Alpha	Beta
Mean Age in Years	52.8	50.4
Sex		
Female	39%	43%
Male	61%	57%
Household Income		
$0 - 9,999	31%	28%
$10,000 - 19,999	26%	28%
$20,000 - 29,999	30%	21%
Over $30,000	13%	21%
Mean Years Education	11.2	12.4
Mean Years Residence	29.9	24.7
Race		
Black	14%	6%
White	84%	92%
Other	2%	1%
Occupation, Head of Household		
Retired	26%	26%
Professional & Technical	13%	25%
Administrative & Managerial	15%	16%
Clerical & Sales	7%	6%
Machine Trades	9%	4%
Agriculture	3%	6%
Structural	4%	6%
Forestry	9%	4%
Other	14%	7%

Effects of Income, Race, Sex and Length of Residence on Community Attitudes. In order to examine the effects of selected personal characteristics of the residents with the responses offered, the variables were cross-tabulated and subjected to the chi-square test of significance.

Household income analysis showed that residents with higher incomes were more likely to rate Alpha above average in solving problems than those with low and moderate incomes ($X^2 = 9.48$, p = .05). This relationship was not significant in Beta ($X^2 = 3.9$, p = .42).

The response rate of black residents in both communities was smaller than their distribution in the population. Blacks in Alpha were more likely to rank their community below average (38%) in problem-solving ability than were whites (21%). Black residents in Alpha also listed fewer community successes than did white residents ($X^2 = 31.8$, p = .004). In general, the Beta respondents showed less difference between the races in their attitude toward their community.

Male/female responses showed no significant attitudinal differences in the two communities.

Length of residence was studied by dividing the respondents into two groups, *newcomers* (less than 10 years residence in the community) and *oldtimers* (10 years or more). Newcomers in both towns were likely to have higher incomes and more education. Alpha newcomers were less likely to purchase goods and services in their town than oldtimers, but the differences were not significant in Beta.

The second community study showed only small differences between Alpha and Beta with respect to the distribution of power and residents' identification with their community. There was a significant difference, however, in residents' assessment of their community's ability to solve problems. Regardless of their race, sex, income or length of residence, Beta residents rated their town significantly higher in its ability to solve community-wide problems. This second community study, like the first, lends support to the belief that the ability of a community to attract physicians is closely related to the ability of that community to confront problems and take necessary action.

Section II.
Strategies for Solution

Many different approaches were being tried across the United States in the late 1960's and early 1970's to improve rural health care. Perhaps most in vogue at the time was development of the "physician-extender," a concept which had sprung out of the military experiences of World War II. These medical corpsmen had the advantage that they could be taught in short, intensive training courses how to respond to special limited illnesses or emergency health problems. It seemed logical that if properly trained physicians could no longer be attracted to the small towns to practice, a substitute would have to be developed.

Even though the rural medical care needs were quite serious in Arkansas, the state elected not to pursue that option. Section II explores the general background of developing the state strategy of approach and some of the efforts that were made.

The potential avenues for increasing the number of new physicians who will live and practice in rural areas can be clustered into four general program areas:

1) The **admission process** offers an opportunity to bring a more receptive or responsive student into the medical educational system. A portion of Chapter 6 will explore some approaches to change in this realm.

2) The **medical school curriculum** itself might be changed in some manner to facilitate the general career decisions, broad skills and special attitudes that are desirable for rural practice. Chapter 7 reviews the critical issues in considering a change in the curriculum and Chapters 8 and 9 look at some of the specific and important features of on-site learning, such as the Rural Preceptorships program and the Area Health Education Centers program.

3) The **postdoctoral years of education** offer an additional opportunity to shape physician interests and skills in ways that facilitate rural practice. The AHECs have a major role in training family doctors for rural communities, and the bulk of Chapter 9 will

review these experiences. Chapter 10 sets out the dynamics of developing a Family Medicine residency program, and Chapter 11 documents a pilot program for training refugee Vietnamese physicians to practice in rural communities.

4) A number of **placement and support systems** can be designed to promote rural recruitment and retention. Chapter 12 outlines several of the placement and community liaison options which were made available in the Arkansas Program, Chapter 13 underscores the critical nature of the University's continuing education and communications outreach activities, and Chapter 14 reviews an experience in health promotion for a total community.

Chapter 6
First Responses by the College of Medicine
by Thomas Allen Bruce, M.D.

. . .there can be no doubt about the importance of good health in the maintenance of personal happiness and community progress. There can also be no doubt about the essentiality of good medical care within a modern standard of living. Regardless of the rate of occurrence of disease in a population, modern social policy demands the provision of scientific and humane medical service to cope with it.

. . . Milton I. Roemer, 1976.

When loan forgiveness programs have been instituted without any other strategies, the results have been dismal. But when they have been combined with other efforts, such as careful selection of candidates who are motivated to work in the areas of need, specially designed teaching experiences, and counseling and placement services, they have been quite successful.

. . . Southern Regional Education Board, 1983.

It is surprising in retrospect that the state of Arkansas did not respond more aggressively in the 1965-1970 years to broaden the base of physician-extenders at a time of serious and widespread doctor shortages. If not a premeditated decision, it at least was a fortuitous one. One concern of many American health planners in 1984 is how to utilize some of the extenders who have been produced in great numbers, and how to phase back their educational programs now that an adequate supply of physicians is at hand.

The problem of extenders, if there is one, is more one of a scale than of concept. The health care "team" is an established and important reality. Several disciplines are needed to provide optimal care, and many clinical activities can be carried out better and at lower cost by health professionals other than physicians. During the difficult shortage years some of these team members moved outside their customary disciplinary roles to become physician-substitutes, and it is these individuals who will be most vulnerable to the expanded supply of new doctors. The goal in planning should be that of producing a proper *balance* between the number of physicians and of other health team members.

In Arkansas the legislature made two important decisions which set the stage for what followed: after much debate and deliberation about establishing another medical school, one which would be charged to produce primary care physicians, the legislators decided to expand the existing school, fund a new Department of Family Practice, and develop a statewide AHEC system. In a second decision they opted for a broadened and enriched clinical nursing curriculum rather than initiating new physician-assistant or physician-associate training programs. The reasons for their decisions were in part political and unquestionably they were in part fiscal, but in an absolute sense they were quite logical. Deciding to create a new medical school would have necessitated choosing a site. No logical site was apparent in a quite rural state; there was no one city which already had clinical facilities adequate to become the base for an academic program. On the other hand, the AHEC concept allowed several towns to participate in the University's medical education programs at a much lower cost to the taxpayers. If the medical school would act responsibly, the doctor shortage could be abated.

The decision about training clinical nurse specialists and nurse practitioners came as a recommendation to the legislators without strong concensus. The nurses were of course excited and pleased to be able to upgrade their professional standing. The physicians generally had considered nurses as their allies and partners, and in large part they trusted the nurses' intentions and respected their ability to cooperate in team decisions. In contrast, they did not know how the members of the new physician-assistant profession would function in isolated areas with scarce resources, and in particular they were concerned with issues of failure to communicate, *independent* practice style, and a possible reticence to work cooperatively with other existing professionals and health care systems. The legislators could also see the validity of modifying one or two of the existing schools of nursing to the new function, rather than

70

starting from the beginning.

The medical school had its hands full. Without doubt there was need to broaden the scope of medical education and to train more primary physicians. Instruction in medical team care, multidisciplinary health care, and a spectrum of outreach programs was inevitable if the goals were to be reached. Highlights of some of the new programs launched in 1974 to address the need for improved rural health care are listed below, with brief comments.

1. **The College of Medicine** made a commitment to become involved in rural medicine issues. Matters of physician recruitment and retention in small towns became frequent discussion topics among the faculty and within student groups. Student newspaper editorials (see Table 6.1), releases to the public press and speeches to a variety of audiences concerning rural health problems were planned and implemented. At a general medical faculty retreat a decision was reached to "educate the numbers and kinds of physicians that Arkansas needs," with recognition that *kinds* meant doctors who had acquired the broad skills and the proper attitudes to practice in a small town environment.

TABLE 6.1
"Dean's Column" Student Newspaper
Editorials about Rural Health Issues

"What Becomes of Grads? The Arkansas Story," *The Medico*, September 1976.

"Doctors for Rural Arkansas," *The Medico*, January 1977.

"Choice of Medical Career," *The Medico*, May 1977.

"Bravo! Primary Care Selective," *The Medico*, September 1978.

"Rural Health Clinics: the Need for Progressive Medical Leadership," *The Medico*, December 1979.

"Graduate Medical Education National Advisory Commission," *The Medico*, October 1980.

"The College of Medicine has Three Major Missions," *The Medico*, November 1980.

"Where Have All the Doctors Gone?" *The Medico*, September 1981.

2. **The Medical Admissions Committee** was charged to review small town/rural applicants with special interest in view of the fact that medical graduates tend to return to communities similar to their own hometown for practice. The Committee used the general guideline that, given two applicants with equal credentials for a seat in the freshman class, one rural and the other

71

urban, the rural applicant should be given preference for admission. An analysis of the five-year period prior to 1974 showed that, of approximately 450 total medical students in any given year, about one-fourth (24.3%) were from towns smaller than 6,000 population, half were from towns of intermediate size and one-fourth were from the "big three" cities;* no out-of-state residents were selected. For the five-year period *after the rural emphasis* admissions guidelines were implemented, the proportion of the class from towns under 6,000 population continued at the same level (25%) even though there was a 14% average increase in admissions. The general distribution of medical student counties of origin for the 1983-84 class is shown in Figure 6.A. It would appear, therefore, that the rural admissions effort was successful at least in maintaining a rural contingent of medical students in the face of increasing urbanization and competition for positions.

Home County Origin of Students
College of Medicine
1983 - 1984

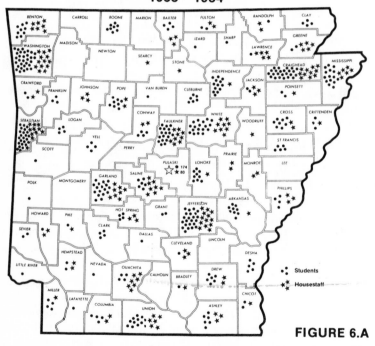

FIGURE 6.A

*1980 census population: Little Rock, 158,461; Fort Smith, 71, 626; North Little Rock, 64, 288.

72

3. **The faculty in the Department of Family and Community Medicine** was used more for early contact with freshman medical students. It was the concensus that if family practice was the single medical specialty most needed in Arkansas, family physicians should play a much greater *role model* function, and the earlier in the medical curriculum the more effective it likely would be. Attempts were made to recruit additional faculty members in Family Medicine, and to make them more visibly involved in first-year courses such as "Patient Interviewing," "Introduction to the Patient" and "Behavioral Science." A more complete survey of the contributions of the Department of Family Medicine can be found in Chapter 10.

4. **Additional high-quality clinical elective courses** were added in the primary care disciplines, particularly for the senior year. Eighty-four new courses were designed by the faculty to offer optional clinical education in general medical specialties at the University Medical Center or at the six regional AHECs.

5. **The statewide Rural Preceptorship Program** was revised considerably and was moved from the senior medical year to the summer preceding the Junior Clerkships year. It thus became the *introductory* clerkship and is believed to have had a very real influence on student career choice, and perhaps even on their practice site decisions. The program has been sufficiently important that a chapter is devoted to its characteristics in this book (Chapter 8).

6. **An increasing use of the AHEC programs** for senior student teaching has been achieved. This had two beneficial effects other than the *primary care* educational thrust listed above (item 4): it has removed medical students from the layered hierarchy of the University medical campus, giving them a more tailored and individualized learning experience in a setting which is practice-oriented, and it has placed them in more immediate contact with Family Medicine residents than would have been possible in the University Medical Center. The dispersion of the members of the senior class also has freed the full-time Medical Center faculty from some of their previous teaching obligations and has given them additional time to devote to the all-important introductory clerkships and to their own medical/surgical specialty courses.

7. **The number of primary care postdoctoral (intern-resident) training positions** has been increased. This may have been the single most effective step of all the activities listed herein. In the 1950's only 20 to 30 total internships were available in the entire state; with 90 to 100 medical graduates each year, it is obvious that the majority had to go out of state for residency education. Most of the graduates who had housestaff training in other states never

returned to Arkansas for medical practice. In 1974 it became a goal to have the number of state internships equal to the number of state medical graduates, and although that goal has never been achieved in an absolute sense, much headway has been made. Figure 6.B shows in particular the expansion of the primary care residency programs. It should be noted that Obstetrics-Gynecology and other general specialty careers have not been included in these *primary care* calculations.

8. **An Office of Rural Medical Affairs** was established in 1976 in the Division of Rural Medical Development with Dr. Ben N. Saltzman as Director. Dr. Saltzman's credibility with state physicians was excellent since he had served as President of the Arkansas Medical Society in 1974-75, and his visibility with the College faculty, students and housestaff was strong, having served as Chairman of the Department of Family Medicine from 1975-77. The Office of Rural Medical Affairs coordinated all outreach programs with state physicians in much the same way that the Office of Community Medical Affairs coordinated the outreach efforts with lay community organizations. The Office also was much involved in the Rural Preceptorship program, in Continuing Physician Education activities and in developing a series of Rural Health Conferences. The Office was terminated in 1981 when Dr. Saltzman was appointed by the Governor to become Director of the State Health Department.

9. **An Office of Research** was established in 1975 in the Division of Rural Medical Development, headed by W. Richard Norton, who previously had served as a research social scientist in the Department of Human Services. Most of the original research studies reported in this book have stemmed from the spectrum of investigative studies launched from that Office.

10. **An Office of Community Medical Affairs** was inaugurated as a part of the Division in 1975 to serve as a bridge between medical students/housestaff interested in placement matters, and of Arkansas towns interested in recruitment. John William North was given responsibility for developing the new program because of his knowledge of the state and his leadership characteristics after having served for twenty years as Director of the Arkansas Heart Association. Chapter 12 in this book depicts some of the activities of this Office.

11. **A new Ambulatory Care Center** was constructed on the University Medical Center campus with a design which allowed multiple small outpatient care modules, each with a different teaching emphasis in comprehensive team care of the type that might well be transposed to a rural or small town setting. This

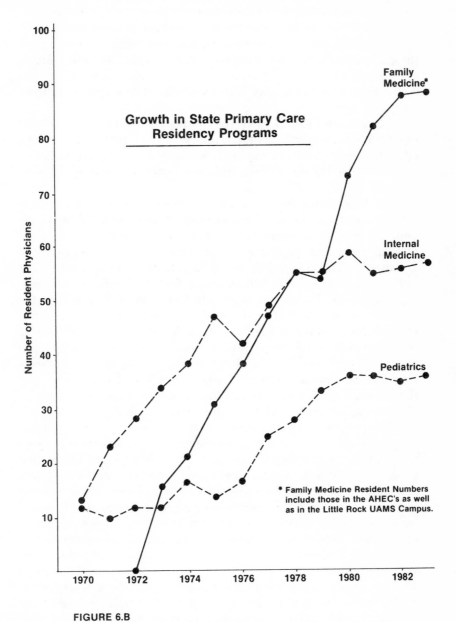

Growth in State Primary Care Residency Programs

* Family Medicine Resident Numbers include those in the AHEC's as well as in the Little Rock UAMS Campus.

FIGURE 6.B

Ambulatory Care Center, after five years experience, has played a smaller role in the rural development program than was envisioned at the beginning, largely because most of the clinical care modules were used by the faculty to provide tertiary (referral, subspecialty, consultant) care, rather than the primary care programs needed to carry out the rural mission. This was not an irresponsible change on the part of the faculty, since the tertiary role of the University Medical Center is an integral part of its function, but it does reflect the conflicting priorities at play in an academic medical center environment.

12. **A Model Rural Practice Center** was established in one of the targeted communities in the state, with the intent of providing a clinical base for learning medical care as seen in a rural community during the period of residency training. That program is outlined in Chapter 10.

13. **An evening discussion group** of individuals with an interest in rural health issues was sponsored by the College of Medicine and was held on a rotational basis in the individual homes of the most active members. Regular participants were members of the University's Rural Development Office, faculty members from the College of Nursing and Pharmacy, a faculty Health Economist, Director of the University Graduate Program in Health Systems Administration, the National Health Service Corps Director for the region, the Director of the State Health Department and various members of his staff (including the Director of the Health Department's own Rural Health Development office), representatives from the state Health Systems Agencies, the State Health Coordination Council, the University Extension Service, and the University Executive Director of AHEC Programs.

The purpose of the discussion series was to serve as an information exchange center for interagency and interpersonal communication of matters pertaining to rural health and to create a think tank of informed individuals who might become more actively involved in creating an environment for change. The general format was that of a short reception with wine and cheese, followed by a prepared lecture or presentation by one of the members, and ending in a wide-ranging and sometimes heated discussion period.

These evening meetings were held monthly for about a three-year period, but finally came to an end when there was failure to gain consensus on specific intervention efforts by the group on rural health issues. Some of the group wanted to quit talking about rural health services, and *do something* about them, while others felt that the discussion group itself was not suited to action issues because of its makeup, and should continue to limit itself to information exchange.

14. **Liaison was established** with several groups and agencies to plan cooperatively in upgrading rural medical care. In addition to the joint ventures with the University Extension Service and the State Health Department's Rural Health Development Office, the College of Medicine developed good working relationships with the Rural Sociology faculty on the main University campus, the state Rehabilitation Services Division, the Arkansas Industrial Development Commission, the state Department of Human Services, and several of the voluntary health service agencies. Each of these ties presented new opportunities for growth and understanding, and all were important in achieving some of the community objectives.

15. **The Rural Practice Loan and Scholarship Program**, initially enacted by the state legislature in 1954, was considerably revised and upgraded in the early 1970's to complement the Rural Development Programs of the College of Medicine. Prior to 1974 an average of six students per class had been provided tuition and other modest financial support in return for one year of practice (at the completion of intern-resident training) in a rural Arkansas town for each year of support. The compliance (success) rate was about 30%, and the remainder of the graduates who had been supported as students under this loan-forgiveness program paid off their obligations with income from a nonrural practice.

In 1974 the number of students supported on the program was sharply expanded to more than twenty (20) in each class, the amount of loan funds available per student was increased to $5,000 per year (four times the tuition level at that time), and the monitoring of compliance by the Board of Supervisors was tightened. The Rural Practice Board was broadened to include the Dean, the University Vice President for Medical Affairs (now Chancellor), the President of the State Medical Society and several other prominent state physicians. Compliance has virtually doubled over the last few years.

Funds to initiate and maintain the rural loan program were provided by the state legislature. Quite clearly there is no cost to the state for those students who do not go into rural practice since their repayment with interest and penalty charges more than compensates the cost of the initial loan. There is a continuing need for financial assistance from the state, on the other hand, to support the forgiven loans; in that sense, the more successful the program, the more costly it becomes in operation.

In 1983 the Rural Practice Loan and Scholarship Program was modified to allow graduates to serve in a community up to 8,000 population and to loan up to $8,000 per year to each student.

77

Requirements to live in the rural community served also were relaxed in order to meet the needs of physician group practices which served several small towns on a rotational basis. The agreement now reads that

> ...the recipient shall practice in and be available to the rural community for at least fifty percent (50%) of the time and shall be employed by or associated with a clinic, hospital or other office in the rural community that is staffed by a physician at least five (5) days a week. No cancellation shall be recognized by the Board unless the recipient shall engage in such part-time rural community practice for at least four (4) continuous whole calendar years.

It should be noted that the state also has developed two other complementary rural practice incentive programs; one is for physicians who have not been supported on the program above, and who are given a $6,000 annual supplement at the end of each year of practice in an underserved rural community (up to five years). This program is administered by the College of Medicine in order to mesh its activities fully with the undergraduate medical loan and scholarship program. A second program is administered by the State Health Department, and consists of a revolving loan fund of $150,000 to rural communities for land acquisition, construction, reconstruction, expansion or equipping a clinic building to house a rural practice. Loans are competitive and based on the level of need and the availability of funds; interest rates are set at five percent, with repayment to be made within a ten-year period.

Chapter 7
Curriculum Changes for Medical Students

by Thomas Allen Bruce, M.D.

A good education should leave much to be desired.

. . . Alan Gregg, M.D.

One thing seems certain — if we taught and examined less, our students would learn more. If we add anything further to the medical curriculum let it be spare time.

. . . C. C. Okell, *Lancet* 1:107, 1938.

The U.S. medical curriculum does not lend itself well to the kaleidoscopic changes in our society which impact on medical care and clinical practice. It is a topic of much national discussion in the first half of the 1980's that the curriculum is vastly overstocked with highly technical and continuously changing fragments of information. The virtual explosion of molecular and cellular biology, the previously undreamed-of worlds of immunochemistry and genetic engineering, the encyclopedic field of drugs, pharmacokinetics and clinical therapeutics, the intricate details of the pathophysiology of a thousand diseases — all these are superimposed on the classic courses such as Anatomy, Physiology, Microbiology and Biochemistry. Add to that the need to learn the major disciplines of medicine, i.e., Pediatrics, Surgery, Obstetrics, Psychiatry, Internal Medicine, Neurology, Anesthesiology, Radiology and a dozen others. Add still again the need to develop clinical skills and to gain experience in interviewing, physical diagnosis, differential problem solving, use of the clinical laboratory and patient management concepts. Superimpose still another layer of understanding the role of nurses, emergency technicians, psychologists, social workers, epidemiologists, dietitians, ultrasonographers, physical therapists, and the like.

It is not so hard to understand, under such conditions, why adding more layers is difficult and why both faculty and students balk at "just one more course" in human sexuality, medical humanities, ethics, environmental medicine, industrial toxicology, alcohol and drug abuse, physical fitness, adolescent behavior, medical sociology, human nutrition, gerontology, etc. The truth is that even with a 10% paring of the lecture content each year, there is a 15% addition to the base of information that must be learned. The fundamental problem of the medical curriculum, thus, is not one so much of conceptual difficulty or the necessity for abstract thought, but a considerable volume overload. It is the need to learn too much in too little time, of force-feeding to encompass the fundamental base of medical knowledge in four years.

How can the medical curriculum be modified in a meaningful way to complement the school's Rural Development Program? That question was asked over and over of our students and faculty members at the beginning of the all-out effort to train more primary care physicians for rural communities in Arkansas. The answer generally was that anything that might keep the students attuned to rural practice issues, keep them aware of the need, or stimulate their involvement in local health planning activities potentially would reinforce a latent interest in future rural practice.

Medical students have an innate inquisitiveness and a competitive instinct due to the very way in which they are selected for medical studies. The school's goal became that of capitalizing on those traits and the progressive problem-solving orientation of medical training. The instinctive urge of a medical student presented with the problem of "inadequate medical care" is to become involved in the resolution of that problem. For most of the traditionally urban students it became a problem to be solved by hiring recruitment agencies and by increasing the sophistication and financial resources of the needy communities. For the majority of those students whose first interests in becoming a physician were to be like their family doctor in a nice small town not unlike their own, the solution was much more personal — how could they, as an individual, become involved to resolve the problem?

Freshman Medical Year

With this **communication of the problem** concept as the central thrust, it obviously was much easier to adapt the concern about rural issues to an established curriculum and not have to completely revamp the system of medical education. A simplified outline of the first-year curriculum includes the following:

Course	Clock Hours
First "Semester"	
Introduction to the Patient	22.5
Behavioral Science	79
Gross Anatomy	142
Microscopic Anatomy	130
Second "Semester"	
Neuroscience	108
Physiology	163
Biochemistry	
Basic Lectures	77
Clinical Correlation	54

Without changing any of the major science courses that are so important to the understanding of a student about the structure and function of the human body, it was possible to weave into the "Introduction to the Patient," the "Behavioral Science" and "Biochemistry (Clinical Correlation)" courses some of the issues of rural concern. The "Introduction to the Patient" course generally emphasizes the typical experiences and concerns of a patient who goes to see a doctor: the worry about discussing highly personal and confidential matters, the doctor's responses to those sensitive issues, the necessity for being disrobed so that the doctor can see and feel very private parts of the body, etc. The course emphasizes the need for the physician to understand himself, his own moral values, prejudices and handicaps prior to dealing with those of others. Students learn something of the spectrum of skills that a physician needs in order to allay the fears of a patient or a family member, to calm an agitated patient, to ferret out the particular events or signals in a patient's story that could help understand the medical problem. The student spends some time doing actual interviews with real patients, one of the most terrifying experiences of the freshman year for the novice physician.

It was relatively easy to introduce into those discussions some of the special problems that a rural patient might have, for instance, in conversing with a physician from a non-rural background; of reviewing how the inaccessibility of care because of distance, finance, education, language, or cultural mores might induce major changes in the underlying disease which the patient had, or in the way the patient responded to that disease. Parenthetic comments of the instructor could not go unnoticed about the special needs which

Arkansas has in rural areas, and about what a priority it is for the school to address those needs meaningfully.

In a similar manner, the Behavioral Science course goes into some depth about the physical, emotional and social experiences of birth, early childhood (including growth and development), adolescence, early and late adulthood, the family, senescence, old age and debility, death and dying. Here again the use of examples of rural issues, unique small-town behavior and attitudes, the family as a unit and its function in a rural environment, the special difficulties encountered by those who grow up in a social setting with limited educational resources, a restricted workforce, imbalanced racial segmentation, housing inadequacies (or, conversely, the special merits and advantages of a small-town lifestyle) were useful in emphasizing a point and of gaining a broader understanding of rural issues early in the educational program.

In the Biochemistry course, patients were chosen for clinical correlation who in subtle ways continued the theme of rural need: the study of carbohydrate metabolism using as an example a patient in diabetic acidosis who had run out of insulin during the isolation of a winter snowstorm, the study of digestive enzymes using the example of a patient who had contracted typhoid fever from drinking water from a contaminated well, and the study of bone healing in the broken leg of a patient kicked by a cow. Each example became a piece of a larger mosaic, one in which the health issues were identical to, and indelibly a portion of, a serious rural problem characterized by a shortage of the proper kind of physicians.

The curriculum content became part of a still larger pattern which tied the individual rural problems into a meaningful context. Signs and bulletin boards around the campus emphasized the search of Arkansas communities for physicians, student newspaper articles discussed the physician shortages in isolated sections of the state and of the medical school's mission to help, townspeople from needy areas were brought to the University Medical Center to meet with students and to discuss rural problems from their own viewpoint,and weekend bus trips were organized for junior students to view the problem at first hand. Students simply could not be unaware that a sizable problem existed, and that they were being asked to share in its solution!

Sophomore Medical Year

The second year curriculum dwells in general on *abnormal* human biology, as opposed to the *normal* human biology of the first year. The major courses are Pathology, Pharmacology, Microbiology, Genetics and Physical Diagnosis. The same general approach of rural case studies was used as in the Freshman year, and as many of the Family Medicine faculty members as possible were recruited to serve as instructors in the Physical Diagnosis course. In that way they became highly visible role models of the physician in the ideal *patient-doctor relationship.*

Junior Medical Year

The most exciting year in medical school is the third year, when students move out of the classrooms and basic science laboratories and into the hospital wards and outpatient clinics for the "clinical clerkships." During the year the basic disciplines of Internal Medicine, Pediatrics, Obstetrics-Gynecology, Psychiatry and Surgery are encountered, and the student begins to *think like* a pediatrician, an obstetrician, a surgeon. It seemed on reflection that this early separation of teaching into the clinical specialties of medicine was an important feature in the future decision of the students *against* generalist career choices in medicine. As a result of such concerns, the traditional senior year rural preceptorship was moved into the summer preceding the junior year, making it effectively the introductory clerkship of that year. Students during this period are highly impressionable, wonderfully motivated and eager to participate in every phase of medical endeavor. The opportunity to serve in the office of a practicing physician who lives and works in a small town is, to the student doctor, the most exciting experience of a lifetime! At the time of entry into the *real* study of medicine, the experience serves also as a period of rededication and interest in general family medicine. The student learns very quickly about the commitment of time, effort and knowledge that is needed in a small town physician, and the student shares in the daily joys and pangs of all those who are caught up in the tide of human experiences reflected in a doctor's office practice.

Senior Medical Year

The last year of medical school in most institutions is much more flexible than the first three. At Arkansas in 1974 all the senior courses could be selected at the option of the student, his faculty advisor, and the Assistant Dean for Student Affairs, so long as 36 hours of approved courses were successfully completed. Two changes were made within the context of the Rural Development effort: 1) a 6-week required course in Primary Care Medicine was inaugurated, and 2) many new elective courses were added, especially in the six regional AHECs.

The Primary Care course was designed to emphasize ambulatory care learning experiences. In contrast, the junior year clerkships customarily match students with *hospitalized* patients

83

on each of the rotations. Those patients customarily are in bed for several days and available for repeated questioning, physical examination, housestaff "work" rounds, faculty teaching rounds and conferences with resident and attending physicians. Ample time is available for library reading on the case problem, consultation with medical/surgical subspecialists, and working sessions with dietitians, therapists, clinical pharmacists, and the like.

It requires an entirely different order of medical sophistication for the young doctor to care for outpatients. He or she must take a complete medical history from someone who likely is a total stranger, perform a physical examination, determine what previous physicians have concluded about the problem, evaluate whether the diagnosis is accurate in light of subsequent events, determine whether the treatment program is effective, decide what additional diagnostic or therapeutic programs need to be started, discuss the case with a faculty physician (who generally will want to verify any significant history or physical findings), and give directions to the patient what actions should be undertaken from that time forward—all this to be completed within about one hour! It is the educational period when *all the pieces need to come together* from previous courses, and when the student becomes a functional physician in a very realistic sense. It is the kind of educational experience that is at the heart of primary medical care, and one that is very much needed for doctors who will be choosing generalist careers.

The Primary Care course at Arkansas was designed to allow three different options: a) Primary Care for Children, b) Primary Care for Adults, and c) Primary Care for Families. The first option is for those students interested for the most part in a Pediatrics career, the second for Internal Medicine, and the last for Family Medicine. Any of the three courses can be taken at the University Medical Center or at one of the six AHECs.

The Primary Care Selective has the following goals:
1. Become familiar with the concept of primary care.
2. Perform clinical assessment and problem-solving in an atmosphere of patient continuity.
3. Relate the patient and his medical problem(s) to his family and his community.
4. Understand the use of common pharmaco-therapeutic agents.
5. Understand the concepts of quality assessment.
6. Recognize the importance of good medical records in the primary care setting.
7. Recognize critical aspects of the health care delivery pro-

cess including patient access to providers and efficient utilization of resources (the medical team, the medical facility, consultants, support facilities, the community, etc.) in maintaining or returning the patient to his desired level of function.

8. Provide awareness of the importance of health education as a part of continuous and comprehensive care.
9. Become aware of legal and ethical decision-making in primary care.
10. Incorporate the principles of epidemiology into clinical medicine.

The numerous *elective courses* which were added to the senior year beginning in 1975 represented a major advance in our preparation of young physicians for generalist careers. Each of the six AHECs opened "acting internship" courses in Obstetrics, Pediatrics, Internal Medicine, Surgery and Family Medicine. Examples of other AHEC electives were 1) Care for the Newborn, 2) Psychiatry for the Family Physician, 3) General Anesthesiology, 4) Dermatology, 5) Emergency Medicine, 6) Otolaryngology for the Family Doctor, 7) Gastroenterology for the Generalist, 8) Cardiology for Family Physicians, 9) Ophthalmology for Generalists, 10) Radiographic Procedures, 11) Clinical Endocrinology, 12) Hematology and Oncology for the Family Doctor, 13) Special Gynecologic Problems, 14) General Pulmonary Medicine, and 15) Clinical Neurologic Syndromes.

General Comment

It should be evident to anyone who knows something about medical education that there are several popular curricular changes in other medical colleges that we did *not* try to implement. Some of these might have been good options, but since no one school can do everything we deliberately have focused our own efforts in selected areas only. Programs which were considered, and which might have been tried as part of an effort to upgrade primary care education with a rural bent, are:

1. Continuity clinics, in which medical students follow a few selected patients or families over a two- to four-year period.
2. Total decentralization of medical instruction, with all clinical medicine taught in a statewide network of community hospitals.
3. Radical reorganization of the medical college structure to avoid the compartmentalization of basic and clinical instruction. Under such a plan there usually is an organ-system orientation to basic teaching (i.e., respiratory and

85

digestive systems rather than Anatomy, Physiology, etc.) and a universal approach to clinical teaching (rather than Pediatrics, Internal Medicine etc.).

4. A strong community medicine approach to clinical care, with emphasis on cost-effectiveness issues, "team" care, alternative health delivery systems, home care, self care, wellness and prevention, "relevance" and similar issues.

Summary

Changes have been made throughout the four years of the medical school curriculum to provide a broad foundation for those students who wished to pursue generalist (primary care) careers. The prestige and credibility of Family Medicine as a career has been improved significantly by using family physicians as role models for students and by heightening the visibility of the Family Practice program within the University Medical Center. These changes were supplemented with a broad array of *extracurricular* events which kept in front of the students the need which the state had for them as future physicians, particularly for those who chose postdoctoral training in one of the primary care disciplines.

Chapter 8
Rural Preceptorship Program
by Paul Woodworth, Ph.D. and Roger B. Bost, M.D.

Do but set the example yourself, and I will follow you. Example is the best precept.

... Aesop's *Fables*

The most positive aspect of the Rural Preceptorship Program is having the opportunity to finally experience what I have spent years in preparation for—finding out what a real-world doctor really does all day long. It is one thing to read or hear about a doctor's life, but it wasn't until this preceptorship that I really knew why I wanted to go to medical school. It is an understatement to say this was a gratifying experience!

... Junior medical student,
University of Arkansas, 1983

Preceptorship experiences have been a part of the Arkansas medical student's education for years, either on a formal or informal basis. Beginning in 1951, junior or senior medical students were required to take a two-month preceptorship with a practicing community physician. The number of students assigned to an individual physician was left to the discretion of the physician and the location of the preceptorship was left to the individual student. This often resulted in three to five students being assigned to a single preceptor in one of the more metropolitan communities of the state. Over the 20 years which followed, the program underwent various minor changes, but for the most part the increasing requirements in the remaining curriculum resulted in less and less time available

87

for preceptorship experiences. This led ultimately to the program becoming optional (not for credit) and thus of rather low interest to the student.

In an effort to redirect and improve the Rural Preceptorship Program, a retreat was called by the Dean of the College of Medicine in 1976. Appropriate faculty and administrators from the College, practicing physicians who had served as preceptors and other resource persons were in attendance. First, it was agreed that the *goal* of the program would be to introduce young future physicians to the conditions and opportunities for *primary care practice* in the *non-urban* areas of Arkansas. This could, it was felt, add to the number of primary care physicians practicing in Arkansas over a period of time and improve the geographic distribution of these physicians over the state. Second, it was the general consensus of the group that the program should remain optional but should receive elective credit. Third, it was agreed that it should be held at the completion of the sophomore year of medical school. The purpose for this was to stimulate the interest of young medical students toward primary care as a career choice and to highlight the opportunities for medical practice in the small towns and more rural areas in the state.

One of the keys to the success of the program was in the more careful structuring of various components such as the administration of the program, the size of the community, the selection and training of the preceptors, the curricular objectives of the preceptorship, and the evaluation of the program. The program was to be sponsored by the College of Medicine through the Dean's Office, with an advisory committee appointed by the Dean to guide the program. The administration of the preceptorships was assigned to the AHEC Program of the UAMS, with quality control to come from the Department of Family Medicine. (See Chapter 9 for a description of the AHEC Program.)

The curriculum was designed from the beginning to emphasize primary care and to expose students to practicing physicians as role models. Emphasis has been placed on how to establish and manage a practice, and a prominent role has been given to the relevance of local civic organizations and social service agencies in a practice.

At the completion of the program each student completes an evaluation form on the overall program and on his/her preceptor. Likewise, each preceptor completes a form rating the student as well as the program. The program evaluation data is collated and used by the advisory committee in making changes in the program, in identifying preceptors who may need further assistance in their role as a teacher, or in recognizing special problems which the students may have encountered.

We have chosen not to make the Rural Preceptorship a required course for all medical students because that might well destroy the fragile quality which it now enjoys as a personal choice rotation for the majority of our eligible students during the summer. Students still must spend a minimum of four weeks or a maximum of six weeks on a one-to-one basis with their preceptor/physician. Each student receives a small stipend ($125 per week in 1983) to help offset living expenses while away from the medical school; a stipend could not be provided if the program were required for credit. Physician preceptors do not receive financial remuneration; their participation is on a volunteer basis only.

Since 1977, an average of 70 students per year have elected this program, or approximately 60% of the total individual classes (Table 8.1). Evaluation reports by students indicate that the program benefits are many and varied. These include the opportunity to apply for the first time, on a limited basis, some of what they have learned in the classroom over the first two years of medical school. Another benefit is the opportunity to be a part of the physician's practice and to observe first-hand the life of a primary care physician based in a small community. Possibly the most important aspect of the program is the influence it has on the individual student's choice of career specialty. Though it still is early in a student's medical education, most students who elect preceptorships are inclined toward one of the primary care specialties, particularly family practice. Evaluation results indicate that after completing the preceptorship, 90% of the students feel it either reinforced or positively influenced their interest in a primary care career, especially family practice.

TABLE 8.1
Summer Preceptorship Program
(beginning of the Junior Year)

	1978	1979	1980	1981	1982*	1983
Number of students participating	53	69	58	71	48	67
Number of physicians serving as preceptors	45	58	55	66	46	64
Arkansas communities	29	35	36	37	29	41

*The decreased number of participating students in 1982 was necessary because of reduced funding available for the program.

There is an important negative element about the preceptorships: a few of the students who envisioned themselves as interested in small-town general practice were disenchanted with the experience. This usually is not a reflection of the preceptor doctor's practice, but of the overall rural scene: the seeming pettiness of small town life, the routine drabness of social events, the vacuum of cultural activities to be found. When this happens, it probably is fortunate in rechanneling the student's career interests in another direction, for the wrong choice merely leads to serious unhappiness on the part of both doctor and town; attrition is the end result, and sometimes the route to that attrition is the destruction of the physician's career, family, or even of his life. If the early experiences of a rural preceptorship can portray not only the advantages of a rural practice, but also its limitations, it will have been a worthwhile exercise.

Evaluation reports from physician/preceptors also indicate quite positive reactions to the program. The physicians enjoy being able to work with the students and contribute to their medical education. Many physicians state that medical students stimulate them to keep abreast of changes in medical education and advances in medical knowledge, and serve as a liaison between them and the University Medical Center. The improved communications and the opportunity for contact with medical students have produced a considerable amount of goodwill in the attitudes of the participating physicians, and previous "town-gown" disputes have evaporated progressively as this program has evolved.

Though it is not possible to prove that this program by itself has had significant effect on the number of students choosing family practice or primary care as a specialty, or that it uniquely has impacted the eventual distribution of physicians across the state, it is known that concomitant with the upgrading of the program there has been a significant increase in the UAMS College of Medicine graduates choosing primary care. This is especially true of an increasing use of family practice as a career choice. Of 220 sophomore medical students who completed a rural preceptorship in 1978 through 1981 (graduates of the years 1980-1983), 97 (44%) subsequently chose careers in Family Practice, 33 (15%) in Internal Medicine, 22 (10%) in Pediatrics, 9 (4%) in Obstetrics and 59 (27%) in other specialty disciplines.

The change of the rural preceptorship from the senior year to the summer preceeding the junior clinical clerkships has not been universally accepted or necessarily popular. The faculty, by and large, have been aghast that such young and idealistic students are exposed to the "dated concepts, shortcuts and assembly line medi-

90

cine" of their rural colleagues (the truth is that these are much exaggerated, and the students learn more about the lifestyle of a rural practitioner than about the illnesses he treats). The private practitioners, although they enjoy having bright young students join in their practice, wish the College would switch back to senior level medical students who already have some clinical acumen and skills, so that they can be helpful rather than all-thumbs observers. On the whole, however, this opportunity for resetting the student's thought on a general medical career may be one of the best achievements of our curricular reorientation and the Rural Programs Development effort.

Chapter 9
Area Health Education Centers
by Roger B. Bost, M.D.

In Western culture, we have delegated much of our defense against disease to complex health care systems. In so doing we have developed more effective therapeutic modalities but have become dependent on organizations that are often mysterious and distant—geographically and culturally—from ourselves. Rural communities are particularly vulnerable to the uncertainty this situation can cause because their health care systems are fragile, often controlled by people whose roots and orientations are alien to the community. Yet, paradoxically, it is in rural areas, where greater proportions of the poor and elderly populations live, that health care services are most needed.

... Rosenblatt and Moscovice, 1982

The first priority of the 1973 Governor's Committee to establish a new State Health Plan was the establishment of a statewide Area Health Education Centers (AHEC) Program. As originally conceived, the AHEC Program was to focus principally on the state's primary health care needs, particularly in the more rural, underserved areas. The program objectives were 1) to train more primary care physicians, particularly family practitioners, 2) to retain more of the graduates of the state's College of Medicine for practice in Arkansas, and 3) to improve the geographic distribution of physicians throughout the state. The program also was to be concerned with 4) the needs of the medically underserved areas of the state for other health care professionals, particularly those needed in primary health care, and with 5) providing continuing education for physicians, nurses, and other health practitioners.

The first AHECs were established in 1974 at Fort Smith, Pine Bluff and El Dorado (Figure 9.A) because these communities had physical facilities in place and an established community medical leadership; full-time physician directors were appointed at each of these locations. The first activities to be implemented were elective rotations for senior medical students and mandatory two-month rotations for second-year residents of the Department of Internal Medicine. In July, 1975, three-year residency programs in Family Practice received accreditation and were started by the AHEC at Fort Smith and by a newly established AHEC at Fayetteville. By 1976, additional AHECs had been started at Jonesboro and Texarkana, making a total of six for the state. Accredited Family Practice residency programs were begun at Pine Bluff in 1977 and at the AHECs in El Dorado and Jonesboro in 1980.

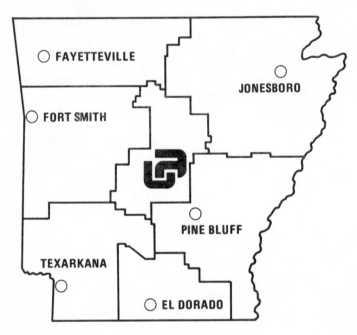

FIGURE 9.A

With its six strategically located AHECs in the peripheral regions of the state, this effort became the principal means of the University to decentralize medical and other health professional education. By providing the opportunity for clinical study and training in settings similar to those in which the graduates ultimately would practice, the AHEC Program offered a sharp con-

94

trast to the traditional curriculum and environment of the mother institution in Little Rock. Offerings were designed to supplement, rather than replace, the conventional educational programs.

Included within each AHEC were several independent units: a professional staff comprised of both full-time and part-time (voluntary) faculty, affiliated community hospitals, a Family Practice Center, other related health care facilities, a medical library linked with the UAMS library at Little Rock, and an administrative and technical staff. Each AHEC is headed by a full-time physician director who develops and administers the educational programs within the respective AHEC. Each of the five AHECs with a Family Practice residency program also has a full-time residency physician-director and two or more full-time physician-assistant directors. During fiscal year 1983-84 a total of 23 physicians and six other health professions teachers held full-time faculty positions.

The AHEC Program in Arkansas is funded primarily from appropriated state revenues. Each of the five residency programs generates income from its clinic practice as a second source of revenue. A third source of major funding is monies received from AHEC community hospitals. This latter source goes primarily to fund about half of the cost of resident stipends. Finally, Federal support has been received at various times for the programs in the form of grants for training in Family Medicine.

Each AHEC is responsible for that section of the state in which it is located. All educational programs conducted at AHECs are approved and accredited by the College of Medicine or one of the other professional colleges of the UAMS; they are coordinated and monitored through a Central AHEC Office in the Little Rock UAMS campus. Participating students receive full academic credit from their respective colleges. Opportunities provided through AHEC courses include an involvement in primary medical care within a community away from the main campus, experiences designed to allow students to supplement their traditional on-campus education in a way best suited to their career goals, and demonstrations of comprehensive and continuous patient care in a private practice community setting.

All medical, nursing and other courses within the AHECs are of the elective type; they include virtually all the medical specialties and subspecialties, with particular emphasis on the primary care specialties of family practice, pediatrics, and internal medicine. Each student works under the supervision of a practicing physician or physician group from the community and participates in the care of the AHEC physicians' patients. The AHEC Director selects a physician supervisor for each student in accordance with the student's request, relative to the field of medicine in which he or she wishes to study during the elective course. At the completion of fiscal year 1982-83 there were nearly 500 community physician-teachers serving as faculty in the Area Health Education Centers (Table 9.1). These practicing physicians participated in all the various AHEC teaching and training programs and were chosen because of their special qualifications and experience in clinical practice. Each physician holds an appointment to the clinical faculty of the appropriate department of the UAMS College of Medicine.

TABLE 9.1
Number of Community Physicians
Participating in AHEC Faculty

El Dorado	45
Fayetteville	88
Fort Smith	146
Jonesboro	95
Pine Bluff	73
Texarkana	42

Following are descriptions of the specific program components in the AHECs:

1. **Sophomore Rural Medical Preceptorship Program.** (see Chapter 8)

2. **Senior Medical Student Rotations.** The fourth year of medical school at the UAMS is essentially an elective one which allows students to design a program of study which will supplement their previous education and promote their future career goals (see Chapter 7). The elective courses offered through the AHECs are intended to provide these students an opportunity to observe and participate in the private practice of medicine as it exists in a community and private hospital setting. These electives range from 4-8 weeks in length and include all of the primary care specialties and many of the medical sub-specialties. Fiscal year 1982-83 records show that 117 senior medical students took 142 rotations in the six AHECs (Table 9.2) Of these 142 rotations, 80 were in one of the primary care specialties of family practice, internal medicine, or pediatrics.

3. **Family Practice Residency Training Programs.** Five Family Practice residencies have been established in the state, in

addition to the parent Family Medicine Program in Little Rock, which is not administratively a part of the AHEC Program. In 1983-84 the five AHEC programs had a total of 63 residents in training (Table 9.3). Beginning July, 1984, it is projected that a total of 67 residents will be in training in the AHECs. Of the first-year positions available for 1983-84, 17 were filled by UAMS graduates and four from out-of-state. A total of 18 fully trained family physicians, eligible for certification by the American Board of Family Practice, will have graduated from the five AHEC residency programs in 1983-84 (Table 9.4).

To date, 166 residents have received all or part of their training in these five programs. Of this number, 57 completed the full three years of training, 47 left the program after one or two years, and 62 still are in training in one of the five AHECs.

TABLE 9.2
Senior Medical Student Elective Rotations

Location	74-75	75-76	76-77	77-78	78-79	79-80	80-81	81-82	82-83
Fort Smith	19	22	20	12	20	13	24	20	17
Pine Bluff	16	19	25	29	29	21	29	31	38
El Dorado	4	2	5	3	2	24	17	8	13
Jonesboro	—	5	5	5	6	21	17	16	15
Fayetteville	—	—	5	15	19	17	25	20	21
Texarkana	—	—	5	2	10	13	14	19	13
Total Students	39	48	65	66	86	109	126	117	117
Total Rotations	47	57	93	87	115	128	160	140	142

TABLE 9.3
AHEC Family Practice Residents*

	Fort Smith	Pine Bluff	El Dorado	Jones-boro	Fayette-ville	Texar-kana	Total
1975-76	2	—	—	—	3	—	5
1976-77	9	—	1	—	6	—	16
1977-78	14	3	—	—	9	—	26
1978-79	14	6	—	—	11	—	31
1979-80	21	6	—	—	13	—	40
1980-81	19	10	2	4	10	—	45
1981-82	20	13	6	7	12	—	58
1982-83	18	14	9	9	11	—	61
1983-84	16	15	11	9	12	—	63

*Figures indicate the number of residents beginning the year.

97

TABLE 9.4
AHEC Family Practice Residents by Year — 1983-84

	1st Year	2nd Year	3rd Year	Total
Fort Smith	4	6	6	16
Pine Bluff	5	5	5	15
El Dorado	4	5	2	11
Fayetteville	4	4	4	12
Jonesboro	4	4	1	9
Total	**21**	**24**	**18**	**63**

4. **Other Residency Programs**. Elective clinical rotations are provided in the AHECs for UAMS residents based in Little Rock; the most popular rotations are those in internal medicine, pediatrics, obstetrics and orthopaedic surgery.

5. **Nursing Student Rotations**. During the past six years, 61 senior students of the College of Nursing have taken three months or more of clinical training in one of the AHECs (Table 9.5). Of the 60 students in the senior class during 1983-84, an estimated 30 will go to an AHEC for clinical study.

6. **Other Professional Student Programs**. Elective clinical training for students in the Colleges of Pharmacy and Health Related Professions is planned for the future, as well as optional educational experiences for students in the nursing and allied health programs of other state colleges and universities.

7. **Continuing Education**. The Area Health Education Centers provide an ideal way to assist practicing physicians, nurses, and other health professionals of the state to keep abreast of current knowledge and technology related to their professional field. Local specialists, as well as fulltime faculty from the UAMS, present or participate in many seminars in each AHEC. In 1981-82, the AHECs offered 341 regularly scheduled conferences and 31 formal courses to over 400 physician registrants (Table 9.6).

8. **Research**. The AHEC Central Office, with assistance from each of the individual AHECs, completed in 1983 a statewide survey of physician manpower supply and needs. The purpose of the study was to determine the number of primary care physicians in each of the state's 75 counties and to project the need for these physicians in each county of Arkansas to the year 1990. This in-house analysis will help determine how many residents should be trained in each of the AHEC Family Practice residency programs in the years ahead.

TABLE 9.5
College of Nursing
Fifth-Year Nurse Practitioner Student Rotations

	77-78	78-79	79-80	80-81	81-82	82-83
Fort Smith	—	—	—	—	2	2
Pine Bluff	—	—	2	—	3	4
El Dorado	1	6	4	3	5	6
Jonesboro	—	—	—	1	1	2
Fayetteville	2	2	6	3	—	5
Texarkana	—	—	—	—	—	1
Total	3	8	12	7	11	20

TABLE 9.6
AHEC Continuing Education Activities
College of Medicine

Regularly Scheduled Conferences*	76-77	77-78	78-79	79-80	80-81	81-82
Number of courses presented	483	516	461	410	395	341
Total hours of instruction offered in courses presented	487	523	461	410	395	342
Number of physician registrants for all courses	3,793	4,221	3,983	3,541	4,352	3,312
Number of individual physician registrants	377	525	361	345	344	—
Formal Courses*						
Number of formal courses presented	4	5	17	16	21	31
Total hours of instruction offered in courses presented	22	16	60	64	94	149
Number of physician registrants for all courses	103	133	351	180	212	401
Number of individual physician registrants	88	106	—	140	180	—

*The above statistics reflect only those conferences and courses that were approved for AMA Category I of the Physicians' Recognition Award.

Currently, four of the five AHEC Family Practice residency programs utilize computerized data processing for patient records, billing and collections, and for various educational purposes. These systems offer each AHEC an opportunity to do assorted kinds of clinical research on an individual residency program basis or as a combined effort. It is anticipated that all five AHECs with Family Practice residencies will incorporate their practical and functional design activities in a computerized information management system within the next three to five years. The importance of maintaining appropriate compatability of data within and among the AHECs is uppermost in the overall plan.

9. **Patient Care Services**. The involvement of the AHECs with public service is mainly through the performance of patient care. This care is provided by the Family Practice Centers located in each AHEC except Texarkana. In 1982-83 the five Family Practice Centers combined had more than 50,000 active patient charts and an average of 6,000 patient visits per month.

10. **Medical Libraries**. The six AHEC libraries provide not only a major service to the faculty, staff, residents and students of each unit, but to the physicians and other health practitioners of the area as well. Each library is linked to the UAMS library, the five-state TALON region, and the National Library of Medicine in Washington, D.C.; each offers a point of entry into this entire medical informational network. Materials housed at each library include a wide variety of medical texts, monographs, periodicals and audiovisual materials. All libraries have a full-time librarian and other staff members.

11. **Community Relations**. An important aspect of the AHECs is the relationship they develop with the community in which they are located. Without exception, each program is viewed by its community with a degree of possessiveness, yet with a sense of pride in its affiliation with the University of Arkansas for Medical Sciences. These feelings are reflected in the extent of the local community's involvement and contributions of time, money and other support. The largest local contribution made each year is the time and effort given by the practicing physicians who serve as the faculty for the students and residents. Also significant is the financial contribution and in-kind support given for the residency programs by the local community hospitals affiliated with the AHECs.

Each AHEC has a Community Advisory Committee composed of twenty or more representatives from the medical profession, the lay or business community and from legislative/governmental bodies and other groups in the region. This committee works with the local AHEC Director to guide and assist as needed on behalf of the AHEC in general and of the Family Practice residency program in particular. This assistance might be in the form of raising funds for special projects, advocacy for the program's needs in the legislature, educating and informing the various communities in the area regarding the AHECs role and significance, providing a hospitable environment for the UAMS students who come to the AHEC for rotations, and sponsorship of the residents for training at the AHEC.

Outcome of the AHEC Activities

The AHEC Program in Arkansas completed its tenth year of operation in June, 1983. This is enough time for an initial assessment of its effectiveness. Since its inception, the AHEC Program's principal focus has been on the state's need for more and better primary health care, particularly in the rural, medically-underserved areas. An obvious means of evaluating the program's effectiveness during its first decade is to assess the progress achieved in the attainment of the goals stated at the beginning of this chapter.

The retention of residents leaving the five AHEC Family Practice programs has been impressive. Of the 166 residents who have received all or part of their training in family practice in the AHECs, 62 are still in training in the AHECs. Of the 104 physicians who have left the residency programs, 77 are now practicing in the state. Six of those who completed the full three years of training have joined the full-time faculty of the residency programs. Of the 27 young physicians who left the state following residency training in the AHECs, five transferred to residency programs in other specialties and seven left the state to fulfill military or National Health Service Corps obligations. The net attrition to other states has thus been quite low.

It is significant that of the 77 physicians whose practice is in Arkansas, 45 are practicing in communities of less than 25,000 population, and 41 of these are in rural communities of 16,000 or less. Furthermore, 21 of these 41 family physicians are located in small communities with less than 6,000 population. Thus, experience to date with former AHEC residents indicates that more than half (53%) locate in rural towns of 16,000 or less, and half of these are in the small towns of greatest need. It is of interest that 15 of the 47 family physicians who *completed the full three years* of residency training in the AHECs have located in communities of 10,000 or less, and 16 of the 47 physicians who *left the Program after one or two years* are now practicing in communities of 10,000 or less.

Another feature of interest is the distance of the site of practice from the AHEC where the residency education was received (Table 9.7). The trend of the initial graduates would seem to follow a "distance dispersion" effect: 55% settled within 50 miles of the AHEC and another 14% settled within a 51-100 mile zone; thus, a total of 69% settled within one hundred miles of the site of their post-doctoral training.

TABLE 9.7
Distance of Site of Practice from AHEC Base

AHEC	Residents Practicing 0-50 Miles from Training Site		Residents Practicing 51-100 Miles from Training Site		Residents Practicing 100+ Miles from Training Site	
Northwest (Fayetteville)	14	(70%)	1	(5%)	5	(25%)
Fort Smith	14	(41%)	4	(12%)	16	(47%)
Pine Bluff	10	(59%)	5	(29%)	2	(12%)
Northeast (Jonesboro)	4	(80%)	0	(0%)	1	(20%)
South Arkansas (El Dorado)	3	(60%)	2	(40%)	0	(0%)
Total	45	(55%)	12	(14%)	24	(31%)

In addition to the direct benefits the AHEC Family Practice residency programs have had on the retention, supply and distribution of family physicians, the AHECs have had significant contributions to the supply, distribution, and retention of other physicians within the state, and on College of Medicine students other than those who enter residency training in family practice. This has been accomplished through the influence of the AHEC Rural Preceptorships and Senior Elective Rotations on the medical students' career-specialty and practice location decisions. Since the AHEC Program was established in 1974, a total of 773 medical students have spent a part of their senior year in the AHECs, and a total of 620 third-year medical students have participated in the AHEC Rural Preceptorship Program. Although it would be difficult to determine or even estimate the impact of these experiences on the participating medical students, it appears to have been a contributing influence, for the fraction of College of Medicine graduates interested in family medicine and rural practice has increased impressively in the past ten years.

The AHEC Program has provided other indirect or side

benefits worthy of mention. One of these has been the improved relationship and rapport between the UAMS and the physicians, hospitals and the public in each of the AHEC communities and areas. The existence of the UAMS programs, full-time faculty, students, residents and physical facilities in the six regional locations has resulted in a marked increase in the awareness,interest and support of the UAMS by the public and by state government officials. The existence and the involvement of the AHEC Advisory Committees in each of the six locations also have contributed to these changes.

Another side benefit of the AHECs has been the upgrading effect of the educational programs, and of the students, residents and faculty, on the quality of patient care in the affiliated community hospitals; this has been expressed voluntarily and repeatedly by those affected. A benefit of major importance is the large amount of indigent patient care provided by faculty and resident physicians in the five AHECs with Family Practice programs. In each of these five communities, the AHEC Family Practice Center represents a major source of quality medical care for medium and low-income families of the area. These services are provided as part of the educational programs in these AHECs.

Summary

The establishment of the six AHECs has promoted the concept and development of a system of regionalized health care for the state, one of the major objectives of the Arkansas State Health Plan.

In addition to the achievements in primary medical care education and the focus on better distribution of the graduates, the statewide AHEC System has provided a natural network and a readymade mechanism for the implementation of numerous specialized medical service programs which are seeking statewide application.

The application of the AHEC concept has served the state well in its first ten years of operation.

Chapter 10
The Family Medicine Department

by Thomas Allen Bruce, M.D.

*The hardest conviction to get into the mind of a beginner is
that the education upon which he is engaged is not a college
course, not a medical course, but a life course, for which the
work of a few years under teachers is but a preparation.*

... Sir William Osler
"The Student Life"

In the mid-1960's the entire nation seemed to be absorbed in the
dilemma of doctor shortages. Medical schools were encouraged by
the federal government to expand their enrollment of new students
and a number of financial and capital incentive programs were
implemented to stimulate and support such growth. Twenty or so
new medical schools were opened, and graduates of foreign medical
schools were encouraged to emigrate to the United States.

That period was depicted well in a report prepared for the
Association of American Medical Colleges entitled *Planning for
Medical Progress through Education,* issued in April 1965 and
subsequently called the Coggleshall Report in honor of its chairman. The most evident trends were:

Scientific progress
Population change
Increasing individual health expectations
Increasing effective demand for health care
Increasing specialization in medical practice
Increasing use of technological advances and equipment
Increasing institutionalization of health care
Increasing use of a team approach to health care
Need for increasing numbers of health personnel
Expanding role of government
Rising costs

A companion citizens study commissioned by the American Medical Association, the so-called Millis Report, recommended in 1966 that general or primary medical education be given preferential consideration for expansion in view of the rapid decline in the number of generalist physicians and the widespread need.

The general practitioner of revered memory knew his patients, did whatever he could to cure or ease their varied ailments, and provided continuing care through the course of minor ailments and major emergencies. His deficiencies—and they were many—were partly offset by intimate knowledge of his patients, the support he gave them, and the trust and confidence his services engendered. Now he is vanishing. Time has changed both him and his patients .... The general practitioner leaves behind him a vacuum that organized medicine has not decided how to fill .... Many leaders of medical thought have proclaimed the desirability of training physicians able and willing to offer comprehensive medical care of a quality far higher than that provided by the typical general practitioner of the past. The physician they conceive of is knowledgeable—as are other physicians—about organs, systems, and techniques, but he focuses not upon individual organs and systems but upon the whole man, who lives in a complex social setting, and he knows that diagnosis or treatment of a part often overlooks major causative factors and therapeutic opportunities .... Comprehensive care probably best indicates the nature of the medical and health service involved. But *comprehensive care physician* is an awkward title. We suggest that he be called a *primary physician.*

The report went on to say:

Medical literature is full of articles lamenting the failure to develop a substantial corps of well-trained primary physicians. Why, then are there so few of them? We find three major reasons: 1. General practice, once the mainstay of medicine, has gradually lost prestige as the specialties have risen in honor and accomplishments. In deciding upon his own career, the young physician may never see excellent examples of comprehensive, continuing care or highly qualified and prestigious primary physicians. He is certain, however, to see a variety of specialists and to observe that they usually enjoy higher prestige, greater hospital privileges, and more favorable working conditions than do GP's. 2. Educational opportunities that would serve to interest students in family practice and provide interns and residents with appropriate training are few in number and often poorer in quality than the programs leading to the specialties. 3. The conditions of prac-

106

tice for the general practitioner or a physician interested in family practice are thought to be less attractive than the conditions and privileges enjoyed by a specialist .... It is time for a revolution, not a few patchwork adaptions.

Some of the newer medical schools were established with primary education as their major reason for existence. Much of the discussion in the existing schools centered on the validity of general practice as an *academic* entity. Clearly it was a discipline denoting a certain style and manner of *practice*, but did general practice have anything unique about it, anything more of substance than being just a smattering of a dozen other basic disciplines? The issues were not easily resolved, and emotion tended to carry more weight than logic.

Logical or not, unique or not, academic or not, the public wanted more general practitioners, and so did many of the older and more influential members of the American Medical Association and the state medical societies. The politicians picked up on all these sentiments and insisted that the medical schools respond! To succeed in the long run and regain its professional status, it appeared that General Practice would have to become a bona fide specialty. In 1969 it officially was recognized under the banner "Family Practice" as the 20th U.S. medical specialty; a three-year residency program was developed with stiff requirements for Board certification and recertification at periodic intervals; continuing education was mandated as a condition for recertification. The body of knowledge to be learned came to be called *Family Medicine*, whereas the service was that of *Family Practice*, and the physicians who were specializing in the discipline came to be called *family practitioners* or *family physicians*.

Arkansas had tried in the late 1950's and early 1960's to set up a two-year general practice residency program to meet some of the increasing state needs for well-qualified rural physicians. Approximately ten or 15 residents went through that program, which included six months each of internal medicine, pediatrics, surgery and obstetrics/gynecology. The program died because the residents had no genuine home base, no advocate for their interests and needs, and they had no real stature in the specialty departments in which they rotated.

In July 1969 the present Family Medicine unit of the College was initiated when the Dean recruited a family physician just out of a residency training program in another state to begin the planning of a similar program in Arkansas. During that initial year of planning and conceptual development an application for residency approval was submitted; provisional accreditation was given and the new Division was inaugurated in 1970-71 using educational development funds which had been allocated to the Dean from a Federal grant. Plans for a model Family Practice office were developed, and clinical activities were initiated in the University Hospital Emergency Room and in the outpatient clinics.

During its next biennial session the state legislature strongly endorsed this new program and provided a special line-item appropriation for the new group which was to allow recruitment of additional faculty members and salaries for the first Family Practice residents. Money also was included for the University Hospital to renovate the Emergency Suite to provide offices for the Family Medicine faculty and clinical examination rooms for the Family Practice patients. The Family Medicine Division was to be free-standing, i.e., not reporting to any other medical school department, and it was to be given the primary responsibility for running the Emergency Room and the Student-Employee Health Service. In addition, in concert with the Dean's Office, plans were laid to develop special affiliation agreements with two of the private community hospitals for supplementary inpatient and outpatient service programs; the idea was that the great body of privately practicing GP's were located in those two private hospitals, and that they could serve as a willing and able voluntary faculty group, supervising the medical students and Family Practice residents. Having the Family Medicine inpatient base outside the University Hospital was seen as an additional advantage in that it avoided the territorial battles that might have erupted if portions of the University teaching hospital were reassigned to the new group.

The new Division Director developed an aggressive program to recruit some of the senior medical students into a special relationship with Family Medicine. As part of an all-elective curriculum for the senior year, he developed a year-long option that was designed also to count as the first year of a three-year residency program. Time in the Family Practice Office was spent caring for a set number of patient families throughout the year. Mixed subspecialty educational programs were set up to be provided in horizontal periods of time, e.g., spread over 12 to 18 weeks rather than the traditional vertical blocks of three to six weeks. Community Medicine and Preventive Medicine concepts were presented through special projects of health screening, supplemented by conferences and seminars intended to integrate the different styles of teaching. The ambulatory practice experience was set up as the core of the Family Practice education program; it amounted to ten percent of the time in the first year, ranging to 75% during the third residency year.

108

These plans and efforts did not fare well, however enthusiastically they were supported by the medical school and hospital administration. The new American Board of Family Practice, at its July 1973 meeting, decided not to approve the Arkansas plan to amalgamate the senior year of medical school into the residency program. The community hospital arrangements turned sour when the specialty staffs voted to deny active staff privileges to the Family Medicine faculty members and to restrict sharply the clinical activities of the junior residents. The Emergency Room/Student-Employee Health services at the University Hospital were unsatisfactory since they didn't provide for continuing family care which was at the heart of the Family Medicine philosophy; in addition, they required an inordinately large block of faculty and housestaff time and effort for clinical service. The residents had their own source for dissatisfaction; the decision to base the Family Medicine programs in the community hospitals came increasingly to be seen by them as exclusion from the University tertiary care hospital. Faculty recruitment continued to be difficult, and when seemingly competent people were hired they had trouble meeting the standard faculty expectations of scholarly research in qualifying for academic promotion and tenure.

When legislators became aware of some of these issues and the unhappiness of the new residents, they blamed the clinical chiefs of the established medical school departments. Senate Bill 337 of 1973 directed the Medical Center to limit administrators to four year appointments, renewable "only after thorough assessment of individual performance and attitude of the appointee in relation to the institutional goals of the Medical Center and the statewide health manpower needs of the State of Arkansas."

The bill further required the curriculum to "provide appropriate courses specifically designed to encourage and support the educational goals of those students interested in an appropriate education for and establishment of a family medicine practice or general practice of medicine." This bill, although it didn't pass, undoubtedly caught the attention of the departmental chairmen in the medical school, but it tended to increase the polarization which had developed with the new Family Medicine discipline.

A number of efforts were made to address the problems listed above. A new Family Practice Center was developed outside the Emergency Room in a doctor's office building just one block away from the University Hospital. One of the adjacent buildings (Shuffield Hall) was renovated into an inpatient unit for the Family Practice group. Numerous efforts were made to recruit new faculty and residents into the program. A Family Practice Club was developed to increase the contact hours with undergraduate medical students and to offer a mix of non-traditional educational programs and social activities. Visiting professors were brought in to further stimulate interest in the growing national prominence of Family Medicine. In 1973 the Division was upgraded to full Departmental status, and the former Director was named Acting Chairman. It was apparent to all that the recruitment of a senior and credible physician who could provide dynamic leadership was a key to the long-term development of the Department and its progress in becoming a full-fledged academic program.

For nearly a year efforts were made by a senior faculty search committee to recruit a strong chairman. No recommendations were made, and the Dean, under attack from the Arkansas Academy of Family Physicians for the intolerably long delay, offered to resign his position and assume the Chairmanship personally; his offer unanimously was rejected by the Academy in special session because they wanted a family physician as Chairman, not another specialist (the Dean was an internist). In March 1974 the Search Committee was disbanded after the Dean announced publicly his resignation.

Resolution of the Family Medicine Chairmanship was the first order of business for the new Dean, who arrived in the late summer of 1974. Dr. Ben Saltzman, a widely respected rural physician who at that time was serving as President of the Arkansas Medical Society, was persuaded to leave his practice and assume the responsibilities for Departmental leadership; the appointment had the full support of the Academy of Family Physicians. For two years thereafter the Department was at peace and showed progress in a number of areas. When Dr. Saltzman moved to the Dean's Office to become Head of the Office of Rural Medical Development in 1977 there was another interim period under an Acting Chairman, and in 1978 the appointment of Dr. Kenneth Goss, the present Chairman, was confirmed.

With the leadership issue successfully resolved, the Department began to invest its full efforts in the directions of faculty development, Clinical Practice Center improvements and strengthening the caliber of the residency and undergraduate educational programs. The Department's activities became increasingly important in achieving the school's rural outreach goals.

Rural Practice Center

A Model Rural Practice Center was established in DeQueen, Arkansas, population 3,863 in 1970, after a statewide competition sponsored by the Department. That site was chosen because

110

DeQueen was more than fifty miles from a major metropolitan area, had a group of qualified family physicians in the community who were willing to accept resident physicians into their practice on a rotating basis, had a well-equipped 75-bed hospital, later expanded to 100 beds, and provided outreach care to several smaller satellite communities.

The goals for the resident physicians were to gain experience in an excellent family group practice in a rural environment, one which used paraprofessional physician extenders in a constructive manner and which was well integrated into the community business, political and social structure. Another goal was for the residents to learn firsthand the principles of office practice management, including clinic design and equipment, medical records administration, business and financial systems, personnel management, the legal parameters of practice, and of intraprofessional relations, including areas of differing responsibility and contractural agreements.

The Model Rural Practice Center was used for all third-year Family Practice residents based in the University Medical Center, as opposed to those whose primary base was in the AHECs. The program was active from about 1975 to about 1980, at which time the capacity to accept residents in the community was no longer feasible due to changes in the local physician groups. At about the same time the curricular design for the University Family Practice program was modified significantly to complement the AHEC programs, and the University Center emphasis switched to that of metropolitan practice and training for a subsequent academic career. From that time forward, the Model Rural Practice Center concept has not been used.

No perceptible change in the geographic distribution of the Family Practice graduates has been seen as a result of their experience in the Model Rural Practice Center, compared with a prior control period. All residents left the Rural Center with positive feelings about rural practice options, however, and some have elected to follow those options by developing their own rural practice. It is the opinion of the Rural Programs Office Staff that the effort was more effective in retention than of initial recruitment to rural practice.

Behavioral Sciences Education

A hallmark of the family physician is generally acknowledged to be his perception of the patient as a person, a person within a family constellation. The Department undertook primary responsibility for developing this perception in the resident. In a supportive climate the residents were first allowed to become aware of themselves through opportunities to explore their own personal strengths and weaknesses. This growing awareness of self had in the past frequently been submerged by the consuming efforts of obtaining a medical education. A genuine effort was made to develop and perfect the interpersonal skills which are so vital to family practice. This was felt to be an appropriate departmental function since the personal development efforts can best be addressed in a longitudinal fashion throughout the residency. To achieve this goal, an intradepartmental division of "personal medicine" (behavioral science) was developed.

The Arkansas Academy of Family Physicians viewed this particular program with some concern, because they were anxious that behavioral issues not dominate a learning environment at the expense of more traditional medical concepts. On more than one occasion the Department had to modify its educational plan to avoid strong criticism from the practicing physicians who monitored the growth of the Department much as a proud parent might raise a child. The Academy thus simultaneously was both boon and bane in the perception of the faculty members—a help in the political process of acquiring more resources to grow, and an intruder in the efforts to make significant changes in the discipline.

Quality Education in the Various Medical Specialties

The importance of strong rotations in the several specialties of medicine cannot be doubted. Family physicians do not presume to have all the skills necessary to teach themselves and so must look to other specialties to help accomplish this important task. Thus, it became increasingly clear that the training of family physicians was a combined effort of the several departments of the medical school. The weakest link in the chain clearly would have a profound impact on Family Medicine. Sharpening the educational goals of these rotations, coupled with a viable assessment and feedback system, enhanced the quality of these educational experiences. Unfortunately, this kind of refinement on the individual rotations, without consideration of the implications of integration and synthesis, tended to widen the interfaces between the disciplines. Minimizing the risk of fragmentation involved in bridging each interface became a major objective of the instructional efforts. Softening some of the traditional block-time constraints of existing rotations so that the residents could provide continuity of care for their patients in the Family Practice Center was one step. Demands of the specialty rotations repeatedly had to be balanced against the broader goals inherent in developing a truly innovative program to teach Family Medicine.

More was required, thus, than just making available to family practice residents some specific rotational experiences. It required a *philosophical* commitment and willingness to develop experiences appropriate for the unique educational goals of the Family Practice resident.

Family Practice Center

The Family Practice Center is without question the most important element for success in proper student and resident education in Family Medicine, for it is the learning laboratory where the resident simulates, with real patients, a future practice. If the learning which took place on the various specialty rotations at UAMS was to be integrated by each resident, it needed to be done as the resident participated with others (nurses, social workers) in the delivery of total family care in the Family Practice Center.

Three ingredients were necessary for the Center to become a successful laboratory: (1) The quality of the service delivered to patients had to be first-rate, (2) the design of the teaching program had to be well conceived, and (3) the facilities had to suit the function. Each of these issues was addressed thoughtfully and modified as the need arose. Inside the Center, the role of the teaching physician was critical, for he/she served not only as a role model for quality care, but as a means for gaining insight into the special issues of the urban and rural practice, of group versus solo practice, and of team care as opposed to the care which could be provided by a single physician.

Television Teaching Facility

A videotape support system for clinical teaching was developed in 1977. This enabled the teaching faculty to experience and explore television as a teaching tool. The facility consists of an observation/control room with one-way mirrors into rooms on either side. One side is an examination room, the other a room for individual or family therapy. It has been used systematically to assess clinical skills of first year residents, to assess and provide feedback to more senior residents identified as needing extra help, and to support an adult psychiatry consultation rotation which was developed within the Department. The facility has been judged to be an important asset in self-education and in faculty instruction of clinical and interpersonal skills.

Undergraduate (medical student) Teaching Program

1. First year
   A. *Introduction to the Patient* Course—Lectures have been

113

given by two physician faculty members in the Department.
    B. *Behavioral Science* Course—Five faculty members have been involved in the teaching of 24 students in small groups.
2. Second year
    A. *Physical Diagnosis*—The entire sophomore class was involved in the Pelvic Examination Instruction Program utilizing two Teaching Associates (surrogate patients) under the supervision of a professor of Family Medicine. This consisted of teaching of 12 students in four-hour sessions for 13 weeks.
3. Third year
    A. *Rural Preceptorship*—This program is described in detail in Chapter 8. It represents the "introductory clerkship" to the junior year for the majority of all students enrolled in the College of Medicine.
4. Fourth year
    A. *Primary Care Selective in Family Medicine*—Four faculty members each year teach 25 students who rotate through the Family Practice Center and the Family Practice inpatient service.
    B. *Family Medicine Elective*—A variable number of students rotate through the Family Practice Center and the Family Practice inpatient service for additional in-depth clinical experience in the discipline prior to engaging in intern/resident education.

Postgraduate (intern/resident) Teaching Program

The special report and recommendations of the Carnegie Commission on Higher Education (*Higher Education and the Nation's Health*, McGraw-Hill, New York, 1970) had a profound impact on primary medical education in America and in Arkansas, and this was particularly true at the postdoctoral level. The Commission recommended the development of area health education centers at sites distant from the university health science centers, and recommended that these perform somewhat the same functions recommended for the university health science centers except that the education of medical students should be restricted to a limited amount of clinical education on a rotational basis. Residency programs were to be carried out with a small group of faculty permanently located in the center and under the supervision and direction of faculty in the main university health science center (see Chapter 9 for the Arkansas adaptation of the model).

The six regional AHECs in Arkansas had a profound effect on the Department of Family Medicine. It allowed the unit based on the main campus to concentrate more on training teachers of family medicine and practitioners with a dominant metropolitan interest; it allowed the AHEC programs to participate in a flexible educational program that promoted distinctive differences in the rural/urban flavor, the specialty areas of greatest expertise, and the administrative structure.

Selection of Residents

One of the keys to a successful residency program lies in the selection of residents. A program is strengthened by residents who perceive a good match between their individual career goals and the strengths of a given residency. Thus, it is important that the resident selection process reveal the applicant's sense of his/her career goals and the awareness of how well the particular residency program can help meet those goals. The interview or on-site experience is imperative as a means of communicating to each applicant the goals, resources, and limitations of this residency. The better the match between the resident and the residency program, the greater is the potential for an excellent learning adventure.

It has turned out not to be so easy to differentiate the programs on the basis of rural/urban interest. Graduates of the residency program based on the academic medical center campus have not infrequently chosen a small town as the preferred practice site and, similarly, graduates of the AHECs not uncommonly have opted for an academic career or a metropolitan practice.

Arkansas Family Practice Education Network (AFPEN)

The AFPEN is a special program within the Department of Family Medicine, headed by the chairman of the Department, and aimed at improving the quality of family medicine education statewide. Because of the special problems in Arkansas of six widely dispersed AHECs, this Federally-sponsored educational network has been particularly helpful in curriculum and faculty development. The original plan consisted of seven demonstration areas:

1. The prevention, recognition and treatment of alcohol abuse and alcoholism.
2. Teaching basic and clinical behavioral sciences to medical students and residents.
3. Developing models of clinical practice that demonstrate efficiency and effectiveness.
4. Communicating the general and specific concepts of clinical nutrition to family physicians.
5. Implementing an interdisciplinary geriatric curriculum.

115

6. Programming a chemical intoxication-poison control information system for the rural practitioner.
7. Developing a practice management curriculum for family medicine residents.

The overall AFPEN program has been highly instrumental in facilitating communications, developing an information system about state medical needs, setting up policies and standards of performance, and monitoring and evaluating the attainment of educational goals.

Chapter 11
Special Training Program
for Refugee Vietnamese Physicians
by Jeannette McC. Shorey, M.D.

By the waters of Babylon,
there we sat down and wept,
when we remembered Zion. . .
For there our captors
required of us songs,
and our tormentors, mirth, saying,
"Sing us one of the songs of Zion!"
How shall we sing the Lord's song
in a foreign land?

. . . Psalms 137

What I inveigh against is a cursed spirit of intolerance, conceived in distrust and bred in ignorance, that makes the mental attitude perennially antagonistic, even bitterly antagonistic to everything foreign, that subordinates everywhere the race to the nation, forgetting the higher claims of human brotherhood.

. . . Sir William Osler,
Aequanimitas and
Other Addresses

In 1975, Fort Chaffee, Arkansas (near Fort Smith on the Oklahoma border), became one of two major national placement centers for the thousands of refugee South Vietnamese citizens who arrived in the United States at the end of the War. Among the group were about 150 physicians, some of whom could speak a modicum of

117

English because of their association with American military troops or because they had trained at the University of Saigon Medical School.

At the beginning of the Vietnamese conflict the major medical school for all Vietnam was in Hanoi, a school dominated by French medical traditions and systems of thought. When after the initial struggle the country was divided at the 17th parallel, the South was left without an academic medical center. American and Vietnamese officials formed a new medical school in the Southern capital at Saigon. At the urging of the U.S. government, the American Medical Association sponsored several U.S. medical faculty groups in developing the new Saigon curriculum. For example, the Internal Medicine faculty at the University of Oklahoma took responsibility for the Internal Medicine curriculum, and the Anatomy faculty at Wayne State University in Detroit took responsibility for developing the Anatomy curriculum. The net result was that all physicians trained in Saigon after about 1968 were taught under American medical concepts and had a reasonably good reading command of the English language.

It seemed obvious to many Arkansas citizens that in the Camp Chaffee milieu were a number of physicians who desperately needed sponsorship into American society and had the basic knowledge, skills and training that would be appropriate for some of the underserved communities in Arkansas. Twenty* of these physicians were selected to enter a special socialization-reeducation program developed at the College of Medicine, University of Arkansas for Medical Sciences; these were supported in part by funds from the U.S. government and from the Arkansas Governor's Emergency Fund. It turned out to be a much longer, costlier and more difficult project than anyone envisioned, but it had definite payoff for many of the neediest rural communities in Arkansas. The major barriers to achieving the rehabilitation effort in good time were not those of medical science knowledge, native intelligence, or the personal determination to succeed on the part of the refugee physicians, but the persistence of subtle problems in communication and the incredible complexity of the change needed in cultural lifestyle and family dynamics. It is a major achievement by those involved that nearly every one of those enrolled ultimately achieved the goal of licensure to practice medicine in the United States!

*Twenty-one physicians were accepted into the Program but one subsequently was declared ineligible by the American Medical Association because he had graduated in Hanoi from a medical school not recognized by the World Health Organization (WHO). That physician in 1983 lived in Houston, Texas, and engaged in the practice of acupuncture.

Requirements for Licensure

The twenty refugee physicians had three hurdles to clear before obtaining a license to practice medicine in any state. First, they had to pass an examination given by the Educational Commission for Foreign Medical Graduates (ECFMG). This examination is given to all graduates of foreign medical schools and is a prerequisite to any residency training undertaken in this country. It consists of two parts: one portion which tests the examinee's knowledge of medicine, and a second portion which tests familiarity with written and spoken English.

Having passed both parts of the ECFMG examination, the doctor then had to complete successfully at least one year of residency training in an accredited U.S. hospital. The third hurdle was the FLEX (Federal Licensing Examination). In order to fulfill these three steps, the UAMS College of Medicine established a formalized program for review of medicine and English and for supervised clinical training thereafter. In return, the refugee physician would pay back the citizens of Arkansas as set forth in the initial contract of acceptance into the special training program: two years of service in an area of medical need in the state.

First Efforts

At the outset the Dean appointed one of the faculty members in the Department of Family and Community Medicine as Director of what came to be called the Vietnamese Physician's Education Program. A social worker became co-director and the extra-curricular coordinator of the Program, and a support committee was appointed from the faculty and administrative staff of the College of Medicine.

As the College had been the physicians' sponsor, so it became its American family. It is not surprising, therefore, that the Directors soon stood *in loco parentis* to the refugee doctors. They found apartments near the Medical Center for those who had families and obtained rooms for the single physicians in the UAMS dormitory. They hunted for household furnishings and clothing for everyone; some of these were donated by members of the community and some had to be bought secondhand. They were an important part of the early rehabilitation of the physicians and their families.

After the physicians and their families had been provided with the necessities for daily living, they began the difficult task of learning the English language as it is used in this country. Although most of the physicians could read the language, very few could speak it well or understand the local idiom. Prior to arrival they had listened to tapes, received some drill in speaking, and heard lectures by visiting professors, but they had received very little practice in speaking English. With the shock of leaving their homeland in the crushing defeat of the South Vietnamese-American war effort, plus the disarray of their entry into a new and strange land, what little English they had known deserted them. They began to understand some of the local speech only some weeks after they had become familiar with their new surroundings and had made a few American friends.

Realizing all this, the directors of the program spent the first four months acquainting their wards with American customs, conducting informal group discussions and confining their formal tutoring to a course in English conducted by faculty members of the Department of English at the University.

In May of 1976 the group was given its first *Test of English as a Foreign Language* (TOEFL). The results were, by and large, disastrous. The exercise, however, served as a stimulus to the doctors to begin an earnest study of English. Prior to that time they had insisted that if they merely could be given a refresher course in medical subjects, they would be able to matriculate successfully. They also had to become more familiar with the multiple choice form of testing. They were encouraged to buy tape recorders, listen to the radio and television whenever possible and discuss (in English) what they heard and saw. They were given tapes which contained questions and answers similar to those used in the TOEFL, and they were tested from time to time with multiple choice tests.

From February through June of 1976 formal lectures in medicine and its subspecialties were introduced: obstetrics and gynecology, pediatrics, ophthalmology, orthopedics, general surgery, psychiatry, behavioral science, anatomy, biochemistry, physiology, pharmacology, pathology and microbiology sessions were given by members of the College of Medicine faculty. At this time a retired faculty physician was asked to join the program to teach medical English. She later was pressed into service to teach listening comprehension and in June of 1977 was asked to assume the position as Program Director to carry the Program to its conclusion.

In July of 1976 the group sat for the ECFMG examination for the first time. Seven physicians passed both the medicine and English parts of this examination on this first attempt (Table 11.1). Seven others passed the medical portion but failed the English, and one person passed English but failed medicine. Five failed both parts of the examination.

The seven Vietnamese who passed both parts of the ECFMG were ready for the second step in their training and were allowed to enter a one-year flexible internship at the University Hospital. (The University had applied for, and was granted, 20 extra internship slots to accommodate these physicians.) In June of 1977 all seven of these interns sat for the FLEX; three of them passed and the other four retook the examination successfully in December of that year.

TABLE 11.1
Summary: Arkansas Refugee
Vietnamese Physician Program

No.	Age at Entry & Sex	ECFMG Exam Med.	ECFMG Exam Eng.	Resi-dency	FLEX Exam	Ar. Rural Practice Duration	Current Activity & Site
1.	33 M	7/76	7/77	76-77	12/77	2 yrs.	Gen. Pract., Calif.
2.	44 M	7/76	7/76	76-77	6/77	5 yrs. (2 sites)	Rural Pract., Ark.
3.	44 M	7/76	7/76	76-77	12/77	5 yrs.	Init. Ark. rural pract.
4.	25 M (husb. of 5)	7/76	7/76	76-77	6/77	2 yrs.	Re-enter FP resid., Fla.
5.	25 F (wife of 4)	7/76	7/76	76-77	6/77	2 yrs.	Health Dept., Fla.
6.	28 M (husb. of 16)	7/76	7/76	76-77	6/77	4 yrs.	Anesth., Tenn.
7.	38 M	7/76	7/76	76-77	12/77	3 yrs. (2 sites)	Health Dept., Tenn.
8.	38 M	7/76	1/77	77-78	6/78	3 yrs.	Locum tenens, Ark.
9.	26 M	7/76	5/77	77-78	6/78	1 yr.	Re-enter Int. Med. resid., Md.
10.	45 M	7/76	1/77	77-78	12/77	2 yrs.	2 yrs. pract., Calif. & Health Dept., Calif.
11.	40 M	7/77	7/76	77-78	6/78	5 yrs.	Init. Ark. rural pract.
12.	28 M	7/76	7/77	77-78	6/78	5 yrs.	Init. Ark. rural pract.
13.	27 M	7/76	5/77	77-78	12/79	3 yrs. (2 sites)	Re-enter FP resid., Fla.
14.	28 M	7/76	7/77	77-78	6/78	4½ yrs. (2 sites)	Re-enter FP resid., Ark.
15.	33 M	7/77	1/78	78-79	6/78	service abrogated	Gen. Pract., Minn. (?)
16.	26 F (wife of 6)	7/76	7/78	83-	—	service by husb.	Pathology resid., Tenn.
17.	27 F	1/78	7/80	80-81	12/81	1½ yrs.	Init. Ark. rural pract.
18.	27 M	12/77	3/81	81-82	6/83		(Arkansas rural pract. just begun)
19.	37 M	6/80	7/81	*	6/80	pending	Unresolved
20.	22 M	Left program 6/78 when unsuccessful passing ECFMG after 2½ years.					
21.	24 M	Ruled ineligible because of inadequate medical school credentials.					

*Unsatisfactory FP residency 82-83 in Kentucky

121

These seven then were licensed to practice and were ready to fulfill their obligation to the state. The UAMS Director of Community Medical Affairs had sought Arkansas communities that were looking for doctors and took the Vietnamese physicians to visit several of these towns. By means of a matching alignment, both the communities and the physicians were able to receive one of their top choices. It had been the hope that the physicians could be matched in pairs so that they could reinforce one another, but those plans rarely materialized.

Financial support also was sought from rural Arkansas communities which were interested in recruiting one or more of these Vietnamese physicians. It was assumed it would be at least two years before most of the Vietnamese would be licensed and that each physician should be paid an annual maintenance stipend of $11,000 (equivalent to the level of intern salaries in the University Hospital). The plan thus was to find a sufficient number of Arkansas communities that would be willing to sponsor one or more physicians for a period of two years, at a cost to the community of $22,000 per physician. When the physician was licensed, he/she would then practice in the sponsoring community for a minimum of two years.

Contacts were made with several Arkansas communities that expressed a great deal of interest. The plan was for each Vietnamese physician (and, if married, the spouse) to visit at least three Arkansas communities before accepting a contract to practice in one of them. Conversely, it was also planned for the communities to meet with at least three Vietnamese physicians before issuing an invitation. Finally, it was hoped that communities would invite those they were interested in to return for a second visit before commitments were made. This process, it was felt, would lessen the chances of hasty or inappropriate commitments being made by either party and would increase the chances of a successful practice site selection. It was the additional hope that the physicians would voluntarily remain in the community long after their two-year repayment period was over.

Many visits were made and a number of contracts were negotiated; the UAMS Office of Community Medical Affairs (see Chapter 12) ultimately was involved in placing 15 of the 20 Vietnamese physicians in 11 different Arkansas communities. Five of the physicians ultimately chose to practice in National Health Service Corps (NHSC) clinics which were located in underserved communities within the state. It is not surprising that the Vietnamese found the security offered by these government-supported clinics attractive. The NHSC program supplied them with a reasonably well-equipped place to work, a reliable salary, an adequate support staff, all essential supplies and a rent-free environment for two years. The doctors thus had the opportunity to earn a stable living while learning the complex business of practicing medicine in a new country. A sixth physician was able to make a similar non-Federal arrangement with his community, and the seventh went into private practice with the community supplying him a place to live and a rent-free office for the first year.

Continued Efforts

Of the thirteen physicians who failed one or both parts of the ECFMG, one dropped out of the program by moving to Chicago. The remaining twelve settled down to study until they passed. Seven passed during the following year, leaving five who still had not mastered the language sufficiently. The seven who passed entered a flexible internship at the University Hospital and sat for the FLEX at the next opportunity; six passed the first sitting and the other one year later. Six began general practice in rural Arkansas as soon as their licenses were approved. The seventh postponed signing a contract with a community to visit his mother and exiled brother living in France. On his return to the state he obtained a general practice position in a Rural Mental Health Clinic but at the end of one year left to seek a residency in Internal Medicine in Washington, D.C.

With five physicians still in limbo, a second appeal was made to the Governor's Office when all funds for the program had been exhausted, and $52,000 was released for use as subsistence stipends for those physicians who had not yet completed their training. Since no funds were available to cover academic expenses, the Program turned to volunteers for help with instruction in medicine and English. The faculty of the College of Medicine were most generous in giving their time for lectures and quizzes. An English professor volunteered services for six months, and when family obligations made it necessary to quit, two community women set up daily classes, one in grammar and composition and the other in listening comprehension. Under such tutelage two more of the physicians successfully made it through the ECFMG examination and entered a flexible internship at the University Hospital. The final three struggled on alone and eventually were successful, one in 1980 and two in 1981. Two of these have now completed their internships, passed the FLEX and are in practice in rural Arkansas; the third had not successfully completed a residency program in 1983.

Analysis

Of the twenty-one who matriculated in the program in 1975, eight were still in Arkansas in 1983. Six of these were in active practice in areas of physician need. Only three have remained in their initial rural practice site well after their period of service repayment. The seventh was doing a Family Practice residency in the Fort Smith AHEC and planned to return to practice in the state when finished. The eighth was doing a locum tenens while searching for a Family Practice residency position. This is not an uncommon trend, with nearly half of the graduates returning for additional residency training after an initial service commitment; this is viewed as a healthy sign by the Program faculty. There is also a tendency on the part of some of the graduates to move to states such as California and Texas that have larger numbers of Vietnamese settlers.

One physician has not repaid his rural service obligations; he left the state immediately on finishing his internship because of an unstable family situation. Another, while awaiting the results of the ECFMG exam, moved out of state for a salaried position in the prison system and then entered a Family Practice residency.

Three of the twenty-one physicians were female. All three married during the course of their training, two of them to their colleagues and the third to a young Vietnamese engineer from her home village.

Without exception these Vietnamese physicians have proved to be good and resourceful doctors once they were in practice. Comments have been received from their patients, citizens in their communities, and their hospital colleagues regarding their level of concern for their patients. As an example, one doctor was known to drive many miles into the surrounding countryside to get a patient who needed hospitalization, but who had no means of transportation or the means to pay for it. Others have adapted so well to their new communities that they have assumed broad leadership responsibilities outside the field of medicine. The fifteen Arkansas communities served by these Vietnamese physicians are listed in Table 11.2.

This has been a costly program in terms of time and money for the Vietnamese themselves, the faculty of the College of Medicine, the friends and community supporters of the exile physicians, and the government officials who have given aid, but the benefits seem self-evident and clearly worth all the sacrifices. The Program represents one of the high points of the resettlement of Vietnamese refugees in America, and the people of this state and the physicians themselves are to be commended for participating in such a collaborative venture. The medical care and service repayments will continue to accrue to the American people for many years to come.

TABLE 11.2
Arkansas Communities Served
by Vietnamese Physicians

Name	1980 Population
1. Augusta	3,496
2. Clarendon	2,361
3. Cotton Plant	1,323
4. Des Arc	2,001
5. Dierks	1,249
6. Elaine	991
7. Foreman	1,377
8. Gillett	927
9. Hampton	1,627
10. Lepanto	1,964
11. Marianna	6,220
12. Marvel	1,724
13. Parkin	2,035
14. Searcy (relocation)	13,612
15. Trumann	6,044

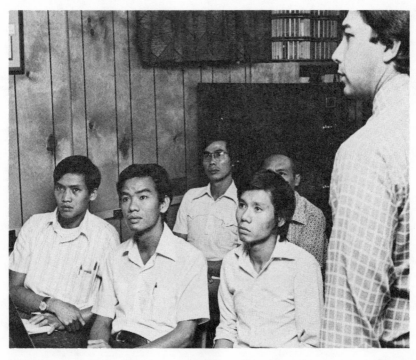

Chapter 12
Community Liaison Activities of the College of Medicine

by John William North

Communities do not have the luxury of remaining ignorant about the intricacies of medical practice. Unless they understand the tribulations and the rewards of country practice, they will be unable to attract and retain people with the spectrum of skills that rural areas require.

... Rosenblatt and Moscovice, 1982.

Building a community-responsive rural practice is endless work, a job that inevitably becomes as frustrating as it is rewarding. It requires a large tolerance for uncertainty and willingness to risk. One must deal effectively and tactfully with a variety of constituencies, any one of which can enhance or threaten the success of the venture. These include community people—supporters and opponents—local physicians, government officials, a hospital, one or more funding sources, a new staff and, of course, patients and their families. Not everyone is enthusiastic for the new practice or emphathetic with its leaders—who are at all times expected to maintain their own idealism, energy,and optimism. New rural health centers are fragile entities, both economically and politically. When they finally succeed in becoming established it is usually because their people—leaders, staff, board members—were as stubbornly determined as they were resourceful.

... Donald L. Madison, 1980.

127

The Office of Community Medical Affairs (OCMA) was established as a branch of the Dean's Office of the College of Medicine in October of 1975 with the general charge to serve as liaison between medical students, housestaff and Arkansas communities seeking to recruit physicians. In early 1976 that informal charge was expanded into a mission and goals statement which was formulated by a panel comprised of faculty and staff from the College, the University Cooperative Extension Service and the State Department of Social and Rehabilitative Services. This document has been revised periodically since that time and the mission and goals statements in 1983 were as follows:

I. Mission

To serve as a resource and exchange of information center for Arkansas communities with needs for medical care and for medical students and physicians who seek practice opportunities in Arkansas.

II. Goals

A. To assist communities, as requested, in assessing and developing the component parts of an attractive medical practice environment.

B. To assist in matching communities with available physicians.

C. To provide information concerning the opportunities for medical practice in medically underserved Arkansas communities to medical students and University housestaff.

D. To assist, as directed by the Dean of the College of Medicine, in maintaining interaction between the College of Medicine, Health Systems Agencies and other federal agencies and the Arkansas Department of Health regarding trends in the health care needs in Arkansas.

E. To assist in making known to the people of Arkansas the roles and resources of the University of Arkansas College of Medicine.

With 74 out of 75 counties being designated by the then-named U.S. Department of Health, Education, and Welfare as *medically underserved* areas and with parts or all of 29 of those counties being designated as also having a *critical* health manpower shortage in 1976, much needed to be done. Additionally, each community saw its own problems as the most pressing and expressed the need for the total efforts of the OCMA. If one were looking for challenges, they existed in abundance!

What follows is an account of how the OCMA responded to the mission and goals set for it, and how it reacted to the needs of the various communities around the state.

Community Profiles

With the assistance of the State Chamber of Commerce, local Chambers of Commerce and the Industrial Development Commission, community profiles were established for all Arkansas communities with a population of 2,000 or more, and on some communities with smaller populations. Information included in these profiles is shown in Table 12.1. Also included was the name, address and telephone number of one or more of the community contacts.

These profiles were made available upon request to medical students, housestaff and any other interested physicians (mostly out-of-state practitioners interested in relocating in Arkansas). Having received the profile of the community in which they were interested, the inquirer had two options: 1) to call or write directly to the contact person and proceed independently with arrangements from that point, or 2) to ask the OCMA to handle the initial inquiries to that community and then, if the reply was favorable, ask the Office to arrange for the visit.

TABLE 12.1
Information Contained in Community Profiles

Geographic location within the state
County and community population
Trade area population and business statistics
Number of physicians and their specialty
Hospitals and the number of dedicated beds
Nursing homes by type and occupancy
Number of community pharmacies
Availability of ambulance and emergency services
Distance to the closest regional hospitals
Availability of clinic space and staff
Availability of private housing or apartments
Educational facilities at all levels
Library and reference facilities
Newspapers, radio/television reception
Distance to nearest metropolitan area
Churches and other centers of worship
Airport/air strip facilities
Civic clubs and special interest organizations
Recreational and sports facilities
Type of city and county government
Kinds of local businesses/industries
Financial and lending institutions

If a visit were planned, the student or physician was encouraged to bring the spouse, and the community also was urged to include the spouse in any invitation.

Students and physicians were advised never to make a practice location decision based only on a study of the community profile, but rather to make at least one planned visit to the community in which they were interested. They were advised further that during the visit, and before any commitments were made, they needed to ask a great many questions and see as much of the town and its surrounding environs as possible in order to be sure that the community would provide them with the kind of income and lifestyle which would be satisfactory over many years.

Resident Lists (by Discipline)

Upon request from a bona fide community source (physician recruitment and retention committee, local physician or hospital administrator) the OCMA would provide a list of names, addresses and telephone numbers of selected interested residents in their final years of training. If the community requested it, the OCMA would make the initial contact with one or more residents. However, it was recommended that the initial communication come from the community source and that the first call, whenever possible, be made by a local physician. It was further recommended that recruitment negotiations not begin until at least one visit by the physician and spouse had been made to the local community, and until enough in-depth questions had been asked to assure all concerned that there was a reasonable chance that the physician would stay for many years. Communities were advised repeatedly to think of doctors in teams and groups because modern graduates generally consider solo practice to be undesirable.

Over the years communities have improved considerably in the way they have used these resident lists. They no longer ask for a list of all the residents in training, realizing that the recruitment of a cardiovascular surgeon to a town with a population of 3,800 is simply not feasible. They no longer mass-mail letters that begin "Dear Doctor," rather than addressing the individual by name. When a particularly attractive candidate has been identified they can launch an aggressive, highly personal recruitment effort with emphasis on a community visit, inclusion of the spouse, and the ability to answer intelligent questions about the town and its medical support systems.

"Another Arkansas Practice Opportunity" Exhibit

This exhibit (see photograph) has been located in a high density pedestrian traffic area in the University Medical Center and has

130

been used to display pertinent information about the various communities in Arkansas which were seeking to recruit physicians. The exhibit featured one community at a time for approximately a three-week period.

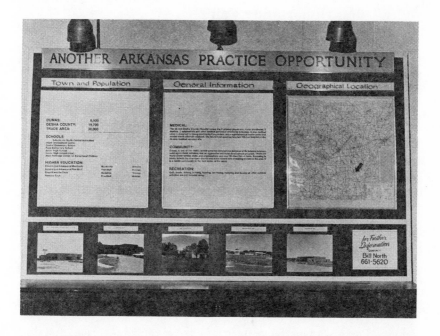

Three panels were present on the exhibit. The first gave information concerning the trade area population, the number of physicians already in the area and their disciplines, the number of hospital and nursing home beds, the number of pharmacies and the distance to the next larger hospital.

The second panel contained information regarding educational facilities, recreational facilities, radio and television channels, newspapers and the distance to the nearest metropolitan area.

The third had a map of the state, with a large red arrow pointing to the featured community.

Below these panels was a space for several 8 x 10 inch photographs of the community and its immediate surroundings. These photographs have been the highlight of the exhibit in the sense that they are the feature most likely to cause passersby to stop and look more closely.

Finally, the exhibit provided the address and telephone number of the OCMA for those interested in additional information or interested in contacting someone in the featured community.

This had not been intended as a *hard sell* recruitment approach for one particular series of towns, but, rather, a way to remind medical students and residents on a daily basis that many good practice opportunities are available in the state.

Physicians Opportunity Fair

The Physicians Opportunity Fair was developed to provide Arkansas communities an opportunity for more direct contact with medical students and housestaff and to provide students and house-staff an opportunity to become acquainted with recruiting communities. It was sponsored by the College of Medicine, its medical alumni organization (Arkansas Caduceus Club) and the Arkansas Medical Society.

The Fair is a one-day autumn event that takes place in the lounge of the Student Union on the Little Rock UAMS campus. A statewide invitation is issued to all communities interested in recruiting physicians, and those who accept are provided with a booth which is six feet deep and eight feet wide. There is no charge to the community, but they must provide all their own display materials and the personnel to staff the booth from 11:00 a.m. to 5:00 p.m.

The communities have been advised that the success of their recruiting efforts will be considerably enhanced if one or more of their local physicians can be persuaded to help man the booth—advice that a number of communities have followed.

Invitations to attend are sent to all medical students and residents. Posters advertising the event are given widespread distribution not only on the University medical campus, but in the affiliated teaching hospitals and in each of the six AHECs. As a further incentive for attendance, attendees complete a registration slip that subsequently is drawn as a door prize, and the student winner and the housestaff winner each receives a dinner for two at one of Little Rock's better restaurants.

When the Fair is in full swing it resembles a somewhat dignified county fair. Medical students and housestaff visit the various community booths, cheerfully accept the various handouts and brochures that are provided, and listen to the story that the various communities have to tell concerning their need for physicians. The use of balloons and streamers, free coffee and donuts gives the Fair a pleasant holiday atmosphere.

Since the inception of the Fair in 1974, both the attendees and the communities have become considerably more sophisticated in their approach to the event. The communities have done away with the hand-lettered signs on brown butcher paper that merely said "Hey Doc, We Need You!" and have moved to well-planned public relations presentations featuring professional exhibits with photographs, slides and film strips.

The students and housestaff have learned not to judge the communities by the quantity of their handouts, the hucksterism of the Chambers of Commerce or the attractiveness of the young ladies staffing the booth. More and more they have learned to ask questions concerning medical facilities present in the community, the types of specialty disciplines being recruited and how well they would be accepted by physicians already in the community.

Properly used, the event is considerably helpful to all the participants. Communities that encourage registration have acquired a mailing list that enables them to stay in personal contact with those prospects with whom they are most interested. Students and housestaff acquire a prospect list of their own, along with thoughts of what each community has to offer in the way of practice opportunity and an attractive site to build a home and family. The most important value to the College of Medicine has been the validity which the Fair has given to issues of rural medical needs and the spectrum of attractive practice opportunities within the state.

Arkansas Practice Opportunities Familiarization Program

This program has been designed to let junior and senior medical students and their spouses make short personal visits to those communities in Arkansas seeking to recruit physicians. The purpose has been to familiarize the medical students with some of the issues of small-town practice, and with some of the problems encountered by those communities which need additional physicians. The purpose has not been to *sell* the students on the particular communities being visited, or to *match* interested students with the towns on the tour. The visits, rather, have been set up as consultations in which the student's advice is solicited how the town might improve its attractiveness to interested physicians.

The community leadership, in fact, has never viewed the Program in quite so narrow a fashion. They are interested in recruiting capable and attractive young physicians to their town, even if it is several years down the line, and they want to put their best foot forward to develop any linkages of potential interest that the students might have. The students, in turn, cannot help but be impressed with the nice people they meet, the sincere interest of the townspeople in recruitment and the very real needs of the town for additional physicians.

The net outcome, therefore, has been something between the

two sets of goals: more than a pure consultation visit, but something less than a hard-sell recruitment effort.

Four events are expected to take place during the visit: 1) Local physicians are asked to meet with the students and their spouses in a private session for approximately 45 minutes. It is imperative that this truly be a *private* session, with only local physicians, students and their spouses present, since only then will the students ask the honest and hard questions about medical practice in the town. 2) Students and spouses are to be shown local medical facilities, including any hospitals and nursing homes, and at least one private clinic. 3) Students and spouses are to be given an opportunity to meet a small cross-section of the people living in the community. This has been most commonly accomplished during the mealtime. The community representatives are encouraged to sit with the students and spouses, answer questions and provide personal views about their town. Business and civic leaders, representatives of the local school system, and a representation from the local churches generally have been included. 4) Students and spouses are to be taken on a short tour of the residential and business sections and the surrounding area (see photograph).

In order to insure that the visit will accomplish most of its objec-

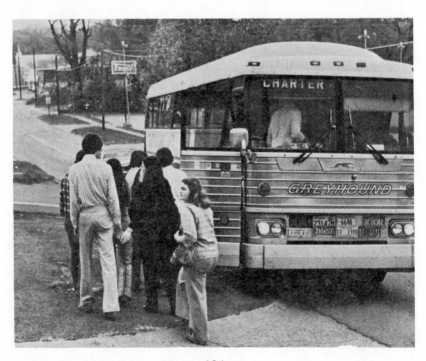

tives, the Director of the OCMA generally makes at least one advance visit to the community to meet with the local planners and help with visit preparations. The local citizens are reminded at that session that the students and spouses are usually in their twenties or early thirties, and it is suggested that at least some of the local group be in this age range.

Several days after the visit the students and spouses have a dinner meeting with the Dean of the College of Medicine, the Director of the OCMA and the Director of the Office of Research in Medical Practice for the specific purpose of discussing the community just visited. Following the meal an informal discussion format is established, and notes are kept on a flip chart of the key comments and suggestions. The students are encouraged to answer three questions: 1) What are the positive things that this community is doing in terms of recruiting physicians? 2) What additional activities could the community inaugurate to recruit physicians (or what are some of the negative aspects of their recruiting efforts that need to change)? 3) How do the students and spouses themselves view this particular community as a possible practice location? This information is then returned to the community for consideration. It is the consensus of the project staff that both sides have gained from the experience—the communities by sharpening their recruiting skills and the medical students and spouses by becoming more perceptive about community issues and health care in a broad sense.

When the program first began, the trips were two-day affairs. The group, with from 8-30 members, would leave the University medical campus early on Saturday morning and return late on Sunday afternoon, visiting three or four communities. In 1982, to accommodate more students with their heavy academic schedules, the trips were shortened to one day, and only one or two communities are visited during that time.

The College of Medicine has regularly paid for bus or van transportation to and from the community and for the dinner at which the trip critique was prepared. The community has been responsible for any expenses incurred during the visit. The only item of any size generally has been the cost of the meal, and it has been recommended that this be very informal; potluck-type meals are encouraged and much of the food is prepared and supplied by local citizens (and it almost always is better than restaurant banquet meals!)

It should be noted that visits are made by invitation only, and that the local physicians must be willing to participate. As of June, 1983, 52 communities have been visited by student groups during the weekend trips (Figure 12.A).

Communities Visited by Junior and Senior Medical Students and Spouses

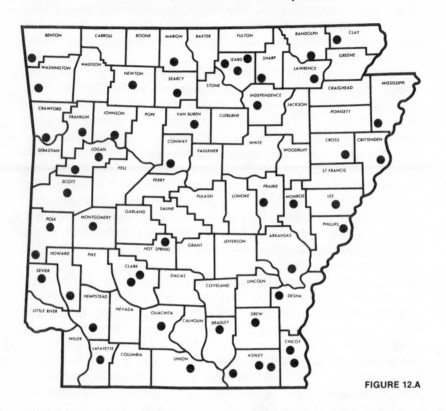

FIGURE 12.A

Consultation and Assistance for Medically Underserved Rural Areas

On October 1, 1978, the College of Medicine contracted with the U.S. Department of Health, Education, and Welfare for a project titled "Consultation and Assistance for Medically Underserved Rural Areas in Arkansas," or CAMURA.

The project had only one goal: To assist those rural communities which had received (or were qualified to receive) DHEW designation as *medically underserved* and *health manpower shortage* areas to define their needs and to obtain primary health care services through a coordinated systems approach.

The results which were to be accomplished by this contract were the selection of at least 20 communities which had the greatest need and were willing to participate in the project. Each community selected was to have the following:

a. An evaluation of the specific health manpower needs;

136

b. The development of a medical environment conducive to retention of health manpower;

c. Assistance regarding the placement of appropriate health manpower resources; and

d. Assistance in integrating health resources to the extent practical.

The day-to-day operation of the project was under the supervision of co-field coordinators, one of whom was the Director of the Office of Community Medical Affairs from the College of Medicine and the other of whom was the Field Coordinator for the Bureau of Community Health Services, DHEW (which included the National Health Service Corps), but who also represented the Arkansas Department of Health. These two individuals were charged with the responsibility of hiring four professionals for field staff, conducting the initial orientation and training of the field staff, and providing day-to-day supervision of that staff throughout the life of the project. Two of the field staff worked out of the OCMA in the College of Medicine, and the other two worked out of the Office of the Field Coordinator in the Department of Health.

In the community selection process, a letter was sent to every town in Arkansas that could meet the qualifications established in the goals and objectives. In this contact letter, the project was described in some detail and the communities were asked to reply whether they could be willing to participate in the project. All those communities indicating interest were placed on a list which was reviewed by both field coordinators for the project in conjunction with the directors of the Health Systems Agencies. Eventually 35 communities participated in the project.

Once the communities had been selected and agreed to participate in the project, the plan called for project field staff from the OCMA to make the initial contact and provide assistance in completing an in-depth community evaluation and an assessment of the primary health care needs. The job of the field staff was not to do the direct evaluation and assessment of primary health care needs, but rather to help the community organize itself in such a fashion that they could carry out most of the work. The rationale was that when the project was over and professional assistance had been withdrawn, the community would be properly organized and able to continue with the development of an environment conducive to the retention of physicians and the recruitment and placement of other appropriate members of the health team.

At an appropriate juncture in the community project, the field staff from the OCMA would introduce the field staff from the Arkansas Department of Health, whose job it was to provide the community with the knowledge and training that might enable that community to take advantage of the various governmental resources available to them. Again, the intent was for the field staff to train the community leaders to become self-sufficient in an area of resource development.

Three special problems were listed in the 1980 final report of the CAMURA project:

1. Recruiting for physicians and other health manpower professionals calls for the expenditure of both time and money on the part of the community concerned. In some communities it was found that the competition for the time of competent civic leaders and the allocation of funds (both public and private) was such that the recruitment of health manpower professionals did not receive a high enough priority to be practical. If the need for health professionals is indeed urgent, then the resolution is obvious—the appropriate community leadership must be educated as to the urgency of the health manpower problem.

2. A rather common problem in many communities was that the leadership of the health manpower recruitment effort held some unrealistic expectations concerning the length of time, the amount of effort required and the cost involved. In most cases this difficulty was resolved by the field staff through a patient and detailed explanation of the work to be done.

3. Some communities were not willing, or felt that they lacked the resources, to make what we considered a total effort in recruitment. In some instances they wanted to depend entirely upon National Health Service Corps efforts; in other cases they were not willing to exercise all the options available to them for recruitment in the private sector.

At the completion of the CAMURA project the Arkansas Department of Health established a Rural Health Development Office which absorbed their original field staff from the CAMURA project, plus the responsibilities of the program. Additionally, the OCMA from the College of Medicine, to the extent that it was possible, committed itself to continue the efforts begun initially through the CAMURA project.

Physician Recruitment and Retention Workshops

As the Office of Research in Medical Practice began to acquire solid information relative to the reasons that physicians made practice site selections, and why they stayed or moved, and as the OCMA learned some practical lessons on how and why some communities were successful in recruiting physicians and others were not, it became apparent that the relevant information should be shared. The vehicle chosen to start the dissemination process was a statewide workshop entitled "Practical Approaches to Physician Recruitment and Retention," and that workshop was held in Little Rock in mid-1978. Funded in part by the Winthrop Rockefeller Foundation, it not only presented the collective findings of the Rural Medical Development Programs staff, but it brought in a number of experts in the field from inside and outside the state.

The workshop was quite well received, and there were requests for a repeat performance so that others from interested communities could attend. As a result, a request for Title I-A grant funds was made for the purpose of conducting a series of regional workshops throughout the state. When approved, the first workshop was held in Paris, Arkansas (population 4,000). In the next three months five additional workshops were held in Clinton (1,300), Monticello (8,000), Hope (10,000), and Sheridan (3,000). Finally, a workshop was held in Little Rock to which all those individuals were invited who had missed the earlier regional workshops.

Following this last workshop a condensed slide-tape version of the workshop was made to be used by communities around the state.

All this activity sparked further interest on the part of communities throughout the state, and the OCMA began to receive regular requests for recruitment/retention workshops to be held in individual communities. Although the slide-tape presentation prepared under the Title I-A grant was used to some extent, a majority of the communities indicated a preference for a live presentation that could be tailored to the needs of their own community and where question-and-answer sessions could be held. Additionally, the live presentations could be tailored to fit the time available in each community. Some presentations lasted two hours, others for an entire day, but the most common time frame was approximately four hours.

Most communities felt that the question-and-answer session was very important because it enabled them to seek solutions to their individual problems. Presentations were made to a variety of audiences, most commonly to physician recruitment and retention committees, but sessions also were held with hospital boards, chambers of commerce, civic clubs, and sometimes to groups of interested citizens who felt that their community needed to recruit more doctors but didn't know how to go about it.

Cooperation and Liaison with Other Appropriate Agencies

Since 1975 several other organizations, both private and governmental, have been working on Arkansas' twin problems of physician shortage and physician maldistribution. It was recognized from the beginning that the College of Medicine would be well advised to maintain close liaison with these various agencies. Three of these deserve special mention because of their close cooperation: The Arkansas Medical Society, the Arkansas Department of Health and the Federal (DHEW) Bureau of Community Health Services. Although no formal organizational structure existed, these agencies and the OCMA stayed in close touch by telephone on almost a daily basis, and informal meetings were periodically. These associations proved most helpful to all the agencies, and they continue to be so even at this writing.

There were four Health Systems Agencies in the state, and contact was maintained with the Directors of each of the four Agencies individually and, on occasion, through meetings with all the Directors.

Equally close contact was maintained with many of the county and community hospitals, primarily through the administrator. Additional contacts were also maintained with the medical staff and the boards of directors of the various hospitals.

Still another agency with which the Office maintained a profitable liaison was the Arkansas Cooperative Extension Service, both at the state level through their Health Education Program and at the unit level through the various county specialists stationed in local communities. The Extension Service understood the local political, economic and social structure, which was most helpful. The OCMA in turn worked with them on their own local projects, including workshops, seminars and high school career days.

Because Arkansas is by no means the only state with physician shortage and maldistribution problems, the OCMA has been in touch with other medical schools and other agencies in several states to tell them about the Arkansas initiatives and, of equal importance, to learn from their efforts to solve similar problems.

Comment and Observations

As with all active programs of any nature, the focus of the physician recruitment and retention program continues to change. Communities which eight years ago had no physicians at all, or were at best short of physicians, have undergone a considerable change. Some of those communities now consider that their efforts have been successful and that they no longer have a physician shortage. Other communities still are in the recruiting process but now are searching for medical specialties other than family practitioners. Some communities are still without enough physicians, but they too are able to see their problems more clearly, and there is a growing sense of confidence that they eventually will solve their problems.

In short, the really desperate days are over. Communities no longer are interested in providing total financial support for a student to engage in foreign medical studies on the rather thin premise that the student will be accepted into some college of medicine somewhere in the United States and then return to the sponsoring Arkansas community to practice medicine (an idea that rarely worked anyway). Nor are communities taking out ads in statewide newspapers offering financial guarantees for a family practice physician who will settle in their community. Perhaps most important of all, the communities have learned to ask both discerning questions of prospects who may come their way and to give accurate facts about their town and the trade area population it serves.

It is the OCMA view, admittedly somewhat prejudiced, that all the efforts of the University in combination with the efforts of our sister institutions and agencies have helped bring the communities to this change of focus. It must be recognized that it has been a joint effort, and that the communities have contributed in great measure. All the projects listed in this chapter in coming years will need to be modified to fit the changing needs of the communities and our new physicians.

The new role of the OCMA, in the face of a national physician surplus, should likely continue to be that of offering information and assistance to physicians seeking practice site locations, and to match expertly the particular skills and interests of those physicians with the opportunities which exist in the cities and towns. The efforts of the office always will be focused and concentrated, of course, in providing assistance to those *most needy* communities which still are struggling with local recruitment and retention problems. The rural community undoubtedly will continue to be an area for need and special attention in future days.

Medical students and housestaff may well need to give earlier and more thorough consideration not only to the specialty they choose, but to the area in which they plan to practice that specialty. Such a process must begin earlier than six months prior to the completion of the residency training, and OCMA has the good fortune to become involved in this process early in the course of medical training.

Finally, a gentle warning should be given to those communities which have been successful in recruiting and who no longer have a need for more physicians . . . don't relax too soon! Towns should recognize that physicians grow older and retire, and that they are subject to the same diseases and accidents that cut short the lives of others. Retention of physicians has been shown over and over in our research studies to be a special problem for small towns and rural areas. It would seem prudent, therefore, that even though the effort may be relatively low-key, community efforts in physician recruitment and retention should never stop entirely.

Chapter 13
Continuing Physician Education and Other Rural Support Programs

by Neil H. Sims, M.D.

The physician's continuing education, whether he is a scientist practicing in a medical school or a general practitioner practicing in some rural area, is largely a process within himself, one he pursues on his own. He may have some help from his professional colleagues in the county medical society or in a research group, but most of his true learning— the part that sticks with him—is what he does for himself, by himself.

... George T. Harrell, M.D., 1958.

The education of the doctor which goes on after he has his degree is, after all, the most important part of his education.

... John Shaw Billings, M.D., 1984

Professional isolation has been identified as a major factor contributing to physician dissatisfaction in rural areas. The sharing of medical information with colleagues, the availability of prompt medical consultation and the opportunity to attend the many conferences and other learning opportunities present in larger urban hospitals is sorely missed by the physician in rural practice. Doctors who practice alone need most of all to be committed to keeping abreast of the current medical information and to maintaining those technical skills which are required to practice medicine of a high quality.

The development of a strong program for the continuing education of physicians was one of four major missions of the College of

143

Medicine, as clearly defined in the 1974 Delphi Study in which the faculty identified this as their second highest priority. In response to this mandate the Office of Continuing Education for Physicians was established, with a full-time director and staff. Its overall mission is to provide "exemplary and comprehensive education and training programs for the continuing education of physicians, with the aim of improved health care services to all people in the state of Arkansas." To this end the Office has set about to develop an effective continuing education program so that physicians will have the opportunity to acquire the current medical information and to maintain the skills necessary to practice medicine of high quality.

The major functions of the Office of Continuing Education for Physicians lie within five general areas:

Determining the educational needs of physicians. This is a very critical function in that educational activities should be planned so as to satisfy the professional needs of the physicians in attendance. The information about these needs is determined from various sources, including a statewide survey of physicians every two years, written comments of participants at each of the educational courses, the frequency and type of problems identified through the "MIST" system (described below), hospital referral and admissions data, and the College of Medicine faculty's perception of recent information which needs to be reinforced.

Course Planning. Once it has been clearly established that educational needs exist in a particular area, objectives for the instructional activity are established and planning for the specific course begins. Careful selection of course material and faculty is critical since practicing physicians, for the most part, want to obtain information and develop skills that are of practical use to them in their everyday medical practice. Of equal importance to the success of any medical meeting is the careful preparation of brochures and other promotional material, arranging for comfortable meeting rooms and hotel accommodations for out-of-town participants, planning meals and refreshment breaks, the preparation of identity badges, and arranging for any special audiovisual facilities requested by speakers.

Implementation. The registration of participants, distribution of badges and handout materials, and other on-the-spot activities on the day of the course are important functions for the continuing education staff.

Evaluation. Of critical importance to future planning is the extent to which the educational offering has met the participant's expectations and satisfied his educational needs. This information is obtained by a questionnaire at each educational course. Other

144

evaluation methods such as pre- and post-course testing are used occasionally. Although the most valid evaluation would be a determination of the impact or the change in the physician's practice pattern which results from his attending the educational activity, such information is difficult and impractical to obtain in most situations.

Information Storage. Accurate records of physician attendance are maintained for every continuing education activity sponsored or co-sponsored by the College of Medicine. Ready access to this information is important to physicians who must verify attendance and participation in a predetermined number of continuing education activities in order to retain hospital privileges or to gain membership in a medical organization or society.

In 1974 the Office of Continuing Education presented seven courses representing 124 hours of instruction; these were attended by 182 registrants. By contrast, in 1982, seventy-one courses representing 459 hours of instruction were presented to 1,656 registrants. The total of all UAMS-sponsored continuing education activities (formal courses plus accredited regularly scheduled rounds and conferences) during 1982 was 1,056, representing a total of 1,477 hours of instruction with 12, 271 registrants. During the same year 1,985 (approximately 70%) Arkansas physicians attended one or more of the continuing education activities sponsored by the College of Medicine. Of major significance is the fact that approximately 25% of these continuing education offerings occurred in the Area Health Education Centers across the state.

While formal courses perhaps capture the most attention in the continuing education effort, other types of educational activities are promoted. A multitude of regularly scheduled conferences and rounds are presented at the Little Rock campus as well as in each of the six Area Health Education Centers. These rounds and conferences are open to all health professionals; physicians in private practice are especially encouraged to attend. Mini-residencies are available for physicians wishing to return on campus and obtain an intensive review of current medical information or to learn new procedures pertaining to a particular medical field. These vary in length from a few days to several weeks. Self-instructional material is also available in the University medical library as well as in each of the Area Health Education Centers, enabling physicians to learn about a particular subject at their own pace at home or in the office.

Telephone Consultation Program. In January 1977 the College of Medicine instituted the Medical Information System via Telephone (MIST), a toll-free telephone consultation service for

Arkansas physicians based on an earlier model program at the University of Alabama. This service allows physicians throughout the state the use of a toll-free WATS telephone line to discuss a specific diagnostic or therapeutic problem with faculty in the College of Medicine. Installation of this service represented a continuing effort by the College to be more responsive to the needs of practicing physicians throughout Arkansas and to improve communications between the full-time medical faculty and the practitioners. Since its beginning in 1977, incoming calls from practicing physicians have increased from 1,800 to over 4,000 per year, many of those from physicians in rural areas. Approximately 30% of all physicians in Arkansas are active users of the MIST system. The system also permits outgoing calls from faculty or housestaff to referring physicians or other health professionals for the purpose of reporting patient progress or to relate diagnostic or discharge information to state physicians about their patients. This service has been enthusiastically endorsed by both the faculty and by physicians in practice across the state.

In 1979 the Office entered into a contractual arrangement with the Department of Health, Education and Welfare to offer 2-week miniresidencies to each of the National Health Service Corps physicians in Arkansas. This arrangement offered physicians assigned to medical practices in small communities around the state the opportunity to spend two weeks at the University Medical Center in a program individually designed to satisfy their particular professional interests and educational needs. This year-long project seemed to be quite successful in accomplishing its goals.

It has been gratifying that, with strong support from the College of Medicine administration and faculty, the continuing education offered to practicing physicians has evolved into one of the strongest and most appreciated programs on the University campus.

Chapter 14
Health Promotion in Rural Areas
by Runyan E. Deere, Ph.D.and Thea S. Spatz

The first step in our analysis requires that we distinguish physician manpower from physicians' services and the latter from health, the ultimate goal. Health is achieved in many ways: better nutrition, better housing, improved sanitation, shorter working hours, and so forth. Obviously, a direct and important contributor to the level of health of the population is the availability and utilization of medical services, including clinical research which may be thought of as 'deferred' services.

... Rashi Fein, 1976

One of the unique and most valuable features of small town medical practice is the sense of bonding which develops under ideal conditions between the physician and the community, with a very real feeling of responsibility and well being for each other. The College of Medicine, in preparing its future medical graduates to use this symbiotic support system to advance total health care, established some model community projects in the general arena of *public education.* The general aim of the model used is to increase the awareness of health issues among the general public and to develop better systems throughout the community for positive health behaviors. This chapter will provide an overview of one such project and outline the component activities of the long-term thrust in health promotion which is still underway in that community.

The town of Benton, Arkansas, with a population of 17,676 in 1980, was chosen as the location of the project, a choice based on the following criteria:

1. Interest exhibited by local people, including local physicians and hospital administrators.
2. Proximity to Little Rock so medical students and faculty could actively participate.
3. Population size of the community (larger than 5,000; smaller than 25,000).
4. Number and kinds of media channels and potential support from local editors and radio station managers.

Initially, College of Medicine representatives met in 1980 with a small group of physicians and hospital administrators to explain the project and to review the experiences gained at a previous communitywide health awareness project in Sheridan, Arkansas (population about 3,000). Following this, and with the support of the Benton medical community, representatives of the College proposed the project to a somewhat larger group of community citizens who were selected on the basis of proven community leadership over many years. The longtime goals which were discussed were:

1. To increase the awareness and knowledge of the citizens of Benton about the relationship between unsatisfactory personal health behaviors and the increased likelihood of sickness, accidents and premature death.
2. To inaugurate a broad and long-term public information program which might reduce the prevalence of risks relating to smoking, hypertension, lack of exercise, obesity, accidents, stress, and alcohol misuse among the youth and adults in Benton.
3. To influence the cultural norms in the Benton community for greater support of positive health behaviors.

Citizen Involvement and Assessment of Needs

Perhaps the most important element in the success of this kind of community project is the involvement of the local citizens. Following the meeting of the small, select group of community leaders and the College of Medicine representatives, a general committee of interested citizens was chosen which could assist in identifying specific areas with which the project would be concerned.

An all-day Health Promotion Workshop was then held, attended by twenty-six committee members and eleven other interested citizens. At the workshop, the group dwelt in some depth about the relationship between individual behavior and community well being. Each workshop participant received a wellness planning booklet which was used throughout the day. Lectures, film strips, and group discussion provided the workshop participants with an opportunity to examine their own individual lifestyles within the context of behaviors known to be healthy, and to make personal choices for change in those areas of individual concern. The close of the workshop provided time for the finalization of plans concerning the health knowledge and prevalence survey which would be given to about one percent each of Benton's adults and youth. The group also voted on an official name ("Health Quest") and selected a logo to be used on promotional items such as bumper stickers. Officers for the expanded community group were selected.

The positive impact of this workshop continued to manifest itself over the following months in feedback comments from committee members during their planning sessions and group discussions. They expressed repeatedly the need to involve as many as possible of the groups, organizations and institutions in the city in similar activities. They also emphasized repeatedly the importance of the communications media in diffusing the central message of positive health behaviors, a portion of the project which has received excellent support from the daily newspaper, the *Benton Courier*.

The third stage of the preliminary work involved an assessment of community health needs. This assessment consisted of two components: 1) a health knowledge and prevalence survey and 2) a summation of the perceived community needs, as reflected in the survey, by a group of selected citizens.

Two surveys were used. The first was a random sampling of young people in grades seven through twelve of junior and senior high school. The second was a random sampling of adults taken from a list of households used by the City of Benton to mail billings for municipal water service. Since this health promotion project was to be a long-term project, the citizens' committee of Benton felt that the surveys should serve as a benchmark for health behaviors and the knowledge of selected attitudes about health among the people in the community which could become the base for future measurements of change. Behaviors included in the survey were smoking, nutrition, exercise, use of alcohol, use of seat belts, smoke detectors in homes, safe storage of poisons, stress, dental health and perceptions of school and community support for selected positive health behaviors. The surveys in the schools were administered by health education specialists from the College of Medicine and the door-to-door surveys were conducted by specially trained medical students working during their summer break.

Once the surveys were taken and the results had been tabulated, a citizens' group met to identify and rank the perceived overall community needs. The group divided into two subgroups, each of which listed a wide range of perceived needs and discussed each need in detail, using a minimal group process technique to prioritize decisions. The three needs which were perceived after considerable discussion to be the most important for Benton were nutrition, physical fitness (exercise and recreation), and stress. These conclusions were submitted to the Benton Health Quest General Committee and reported to the community widely through the *Benton Courier* and local radio stations.

From the Benton Health Quest General Committee eight people were chosen to serve as a Steering Committee to give direction to organizing the public campaign and to expedite decision-making. The Steering Committee selected members and chairpersons for each of the three recommended areas of focus, and each subcommittee worked with representatives of the College of Medicine in planning specific project campaign activities. Through the course of preparatory work over the next several months, some members became inactive and other new members were added. The Steering Committee decided to make nutrition the first priority issue to be launched in the public information effort. Exercise was second and stress management was third. Both the College and the Steering Committee agreed that these three needs were related closely enough that they could be programmed sequentially in community educational activities and promotional efforts. The Steering Committee therefore developed a master plan for staging the events, so that the activities in one group would be begun before activities in another group had ended.

Once the three subcommittees had completed their plan for outcome objectives to be reached and the list of activities to be undertaken, the Steering Committee launched the public campaign in a gala kickoff banquet. Invited to the banquet were all of the various project committee members, public and city officials, selected new community representatives, and members of the press and broadcasting corps. Each of the chairmen for the three priority projects explained at the kickoff banquet the goals and activities for their particular group, and there was much general excitement and applause for the planning representatives. This banquet served as an opportunity for all the people who had been working separately to come together in a large group for an evening, and for the Benton community as a whole to be introduced to the wide range of plans and activities its own citizens had devised. (Figures 14.A and 14.B)

The Youth and Adult Surveys

The two main objectives of the surveys were 1) to establish a benchmark for selected health behaviors and the level of knowledge about these behaviors and their probable consequences, and 2) to

150

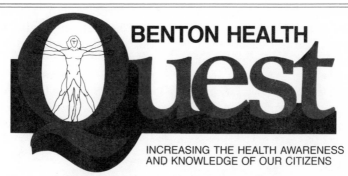

BENTON HEALTH Quest

INCREASING THE HEALTH AWARENESS
AND KNOWLEDGE OF OUR CITIZENS

Benton's Communitywide Health Promotion Program

WHAT IS HEALTH QUEST?

Our health is related to personal habits of living — eating properly, staying physically active, sleeping and resting adequately, not smoking, drinking only in moderation if at all, and managing stress. These have shown to be related to instance of death as well as the **quality of life we live**.

Health Quest is a health promotion project aimed at increasing the awareness and knowledge of the citizens of Benton to the advantage of a **healthy lifestyle**.

To accomplish the goal of encouraging positive health behavior, an integrated program of education and promotional activities will be presented to the community over a period of 3-4 years. This program will emphasize the positive benefits of adopting a healthy lifestyle.

WE ENCOURAGE YOU TO JOIN US IN CREATING A MORE HEALTHY OVERALL COMMUNITY ENVIRONMENT!

Health Quest will sponsor workshops, special lecture series, seminars, and mass media campaigns. These events will be aimed at providing each person with the information necessary for making an informed decision about their own **health and wellness**.

A SUPPORTIVE COMMUNITY

Vital to the process of change is the supportive community. We live in a society that encourages negative health behaviors, such as inactivity, overeating, smoking, etc. One of the prime goals of Health Quest will be to create support within Benton families, organizations and institutions for positive health behaviors. Such a community gives those that are motivated to change, support that will aid them in sustaining their new lifestyle.

RESPONSIBILITY

Each of us is responsible for our own health, and each of us must make our own value judgements about health and lifestyle.

Benton's Health Quest will help you make a conscious decision about your health and wellness.

The influence of health lifestyle behavior changes can have positive results:

EXERCISE
Regular Exercise —
- postpones the aging process
- helps in maintaining normal weight
- increases lean body mass
- increases agility and stamina

DIET AND WEIGHT CONTROL
Maintaining Normal Weight —
- increases life expectancy
- reduces chances of heart disease, stroke and diabetes
- improves personal appearance

SMOKING
Quitting Smoking —
- reduces risk of heart disease, stroke, lung cancer, emphysema
- increases life span
- reduces risk of respiratory illness and resulting absenteeism from work.

STRESS
Learning to relax and cope with stress —
- increases life span
- reduces chance of developing heart disease, stroke, ulcers
- improves quality of life

FIGURE 14.A

151

BENTON HEALTH QUEST

Sponsored by:

Citizens Committee of Benton and College of Medicine, University of Arkansas for Medical Sciences, Little Rock, Arkansas

CITIZENS COMMITTEE

Chairman:	J. Fred Walton
Vice Chairman:	Glenn Ballard
Secretary:	Paula Ireland

D. L. Avaritt	Sandra Krebs
Linnie Bisgood	Donna May
Wayne Bishop	John Moritz
E. F. Black	Colleen Owen
Mike Bourns, DDS	Vicki Petz
Don Brashears, DDS	Rex Ramsay, M.D.
Irma Bridges	Sunny Redd
Clarene Brown	John Riddle
June Brown	Mary Smithers
Roger Burton	Tucker Steinmetz
John Butler	S. D. Taggart, M.D.
Frank C. Chenault	Thomas R. Tutor, D.Min.
Charles Cunningham	Rev. Bob Walton
Renny Efird	Bill Withers
Dewayne Hodges	John D. Wright, M.D.
Lynda Hollenbeck	

FOR MORE INFORMATION CALL:

J. Fred Walton	778-1151
Paula Ireland	778-6525
Frank C. Chenault	778-8326

HEALTH QUEST SUBCOMMITTEES:

NUTRITION

Ellen Cash	Co-Chairman
Clarene Brown	Co-Chairman

D. L. Avaritt	Dean McCormack, O.D.
Gwen Boson	Colleen Owen
Polly Caldwell	Sunny Redd
Jeannie Martin	Katy Welch

College of Medicine Resource:

Margaret Bogle, M.S.R.D., Director, Nutritional Services, Arkansas Childrens Hospital.

EXERCISE

Frank C. Chenault, Chairman

Judy Arnold	Rex Ramsay, M.D.
Mike Bourns, DDS	Mary Smithers
Don Ford	Sam Taggart, M.D.
Dewayne Hodges	Thomas R. Tutor, D.Min.
Vicki Petz	Bill Withers

College of Medicine Resource:

James R. Phillips, M.D., Internal Medicine

STRESS

John Moritz, Chairman

Glenn Ballard	Sherry Johnston
Dot Enockson	Carol Meyers
Jean Foster	Brenda Nobles, Ph.D.
Paula Ireland	Rev. Bob Walton

College of Medicine Resource:

Bruce Caruth, Ph.D., Clinical Psychologist

FIGURE 14.B

152

serve as a social diagnosis of felt health needs. The survey results were used when the Steering Committee decided the three main areas of concern to be used in the Benton Health Quest.

The two surveys revealed some interesting data, some of which was used in the first year of the Health Quest and some of which could be useful at a later date. Some examples of data acquired are listed below.

Selected Health Behaviors

1. Thirteen percent of the youth and thirty-five percent of the adults said they were smoking.
2. Less than half of the youth and slightly over half of the adults reported eating breakfast each day.
3. One-third of the youth and half of the adults reported exercising every day enough to perspire.
4. Nearly half of each sample reported brushing their teeth twice a day.
5. Only one percent of the youth and six percent of the adults reported always fastening seat belts.

Knowledge Levels of Health Behavior Consequences

1. In the youth sample only sixty-six percent knew that cigarette smoking is one of the major risk factors of coronary heart disease, while in the adult sample sixty-eight percent knew and the remainder reported that they did not know or that it was not a major risk.
2. Slightly over half in both groups knew that food attitudes are developed from family eating habits.
3. Ninety-one percent of the adults knew that stress affects blood pressure.
4. Only twenty-nine percent of the youth and fifty-one percent of the adults knew that heart disease is the major cause of death among adults in the United States.

Nutrition: Goals and Activities

Seven people from the Benton Health Quest General Committee were asked to serve on a steering committee. The committee recommended chairpeople and members for each of the three objectives. These objectives were as follows:

1. To provide nutrition information in physicians' offices
2. To provide healthy choices of food in school lunches and school snacks
3. To conduct workshops on nutrition

A major activity of the nutrition program was a Slim-A-Thon which served to launch the entire Health Quest project in the community. This activity was supported by the Benton State Bank (which gave a $100 cash prize and $100 for expenses) and by donations by businesses in the community. The participants received diet information and pointers on better nutrition. At the first meeting, 298 people weighed in and consulting was provided. This first one-hour session emphasized good nutrition. The second session emphasized nutrition and exercise, with eighty-six participants attending. The third session emphasized nutrition and stress, with eighty-five participants attending. The final weigh-out had seventy-eight people who met their one-month contract goal and thus qualified for the prize drawing.

Other activities of the nutrition committee included the following:

1. A series of four articles written for the local paper and featured weekly.
2. Three nutrition seminars conducted by the resource person which addressed general nutrition and nutrition for the athlete.
3. A low-calorie cooking workshop, attended by forty-two people.
4. Ten twenty-five minute sessions concerning nutrition and athletics.
5. Nutrition resource material recommended to the public and available in libraries.

Exercise: Goals and Activities

The exercise committee arrived at two main objectives for its work:

1. To increase the knowledge of Benton adults about the benefits of exercise on their health.
2. To increase the number of adults following an aerobic exercise program.

One of the main activities of the Exercise Committee concerned its cooperative work with the Junior Honor Society in sponsoring three runs: the "Honor Run," the "Fun Run," and the "Parent-Child Run." This particular activity is noteworthy for using the popularity of an activity already familiar to the community, the Honor Society annual run, and expanding it to include more people from the area. The Nutrition Committee and the Stress Committee each set up and manned their own educational booths in the assembly area before the runs took place.

Another activity of the Exercise Committee was a workshop entitled "How to Get Into a Personal Exercise Program." Several runners taught the participants about the benefits of running and increased the enthusiasm for this type of activity. A member of the

Stress Committee was present to teach two relaxation techniques to assist in stress management.

The Exercise Committee also published a series of articles in the *Benton Courier* on the relationship of exercise to disease, psychological benefits, weight loss, youth and the elderly.

Stress Management: Goals and Activities

The Stress Management Committee identified three main goals for further development:

1. To increase the knowledge of Benton adults about what stress is.
2. To assist Benton adults to increase knowledge of how stress affects the individual's physical and mental well-being.
3. To enhance the skills of Benton adults in dealing with stress.

One of the activities of the Stress Management Committee caught the interest of the public through audience participation tactics. A contest was held through the *Benton Courier* in which the reader would complete sentences such as "Stress is . . . ," "You know you are under stress when . . . ," and "You know you can cope with stress when . . . ." Prizes were awarded to the winners. A television interview was also held with an expert on stress.

Other plans of the Stress Management Committee included:

1. Talk on stress and eating habits at Slim-A-Thon
2. Video tape talks on television
3. Lectures to civic clubs, clubs, organizations, and schools
4. Informational workshops involving what stress is, how to recognize it, and what to do about it
5. Skill-building workshops involving relaxation techniques, time management, thought-stopping techniques, dealing with maladaption beliefs, effective coping and communications, and financial planning.

Lifestyle Modification Workshops

An important activity of the Benton Health Quest involved lifestyle modification workshops. The workshop model was comprised of the following components: 1) health assessment; 2) orientation to wellness; 3) decision whether to change one or more health habits; 4) information and reinforcement for the changes intended. The health assessment session began at 6:00 a.m., after a fourteen-hour fast. Physical and written assessments were taken, including multiple body measurements, a blood sample, demographic information, and a health awareness, knowledge, and practice questionnaire.

The objective of the next two sessions was to increase the participants' awareness of the relationship of health habits to wellness and sickness. The personal health risk appraisal results were returned to each participant in the third session. These results were used to assist in evaluating the participant's risk, compared to the average person in the United States of the same age, sex, and race, for each of the twelve most frequent causes of death.

Near the close of the third session each participant was offered the option of dropping from the activity or making a self-contract to initiate a health behavior change relating to diet, weight control, exercise, smoking cessation, or stress management. Although participants were encouraged to work in only one area of change, approximately half signed to start two changes, five signed to start three changes, and one even opted for four changes.

The fourth through the seventh sessions concentrated on sharing information with the participants about themselves. They each tested themselves for balance, flexibility, reaction time, and abdominal strength. In addition, they experienced a relaxation technique, took Holmes' Life Change Stress Test, a nutrition quiz, a daily nutrition assessment and a smoking quiz. All participants viewed films on stress management and non-smokers' rights. An evaluation of the knowledge change showed an increase in the overall correct answer response from 74.2% in the pre-test to 93.1% in the post-test survey. Fifty-seven percent of the participants who completed the questionnaire said they were already in the process of making a change in their health habits when they enrolled in the workshop. Seventy-four percent said they initiated another change as a result of the workshop experience. In addition, sixty-seven percent of the participants enrolled in the fall workshop said they were going to start still another change.

Benton High School Class in Health Education

A less-successful activity undertaken by the Benton Health Quest was a pilot study in the high school of a health education class. Students and teachers in that class attempted a learning activity which was different from that ordinarily undertaken in such a class, an emphasis on lifestyle and lifestyle changes. The goals of this endeavor were to increase the students' awareness and knowledge of what negative and positive habits could do for the individual's level of wellness, and to elicit from each student a personal behavioral change that had occurred or that would be planned. The class was taught in a workshop style with emphasis on group involvement and group activities.

It was the general assessment by school administrators, teachers, nurses, and the teacher responsible for the class that the special class idea was not especially successful in terms of accomplishing the objectives. Even though there was excellent support from the school administrators, the teacher and the school nurse, the students' enthusiasm for participation in the various opportunities was not evident. Their health and learning about health was not a high priority. The traditional pedagogical approach seemed to be entrenched in their expectation for classroom activities. A conclusion reached by core staff members for this activity was that the close association of health education to sports in the school setting does not create a desire of high school youth to learn about the realtionship of health behavior to wellness.

Preliminary Recommendations

The Benton Health Quest has not ended. Immediate participation and successes will have lasting value only if long-term behavioral changes are made. At the end of its first year, the Benton Health Quest initiated activities aimed at the accomplishments of the behavioral objectives.

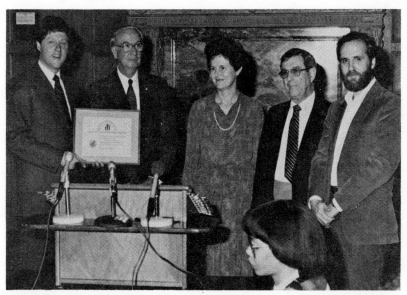

The Benton Health Quest project in 1984 received a special commendation award from Secretary Margaret Heckler of the U.S. Department of Health and Human Services. Arkansas Governor Bill Clinton (at left) presents a plaque of appreciation to Dr. Deere, with Mrs. Clarene Brown and Dr. Sam Taggart (far right) representing the Benton community; Mr. Bill North, Director of Community Medical Affairs at UAMS, stands second from the right.

As a result of its first year, the Committee offered these recommendations if such a project were initiated in another community:

1. Establish guidelines for committee functions.
2. The overall committee chairman should assume full leadership for final decisions about the project in the community.
3. Where possible, persons who have expertise in the subject-matter field should chair project committees.
4. All project committee members should be appointed by the project chairperson. Committee chairpeople should not arbitrarily invite individuals to serve without clearing with the project chairperson.
5. It seems desirable to have an identifiable project office, with a staff person either part-time or full-time.
6. Provision of some financing for the project by the community would probably bring a stronger commitment to the project.

Section III: Future Directions

The end of a decade of intensive rural development is at hand. The final two chapters will attempt to summarize the impact of the activities that were instituted to deal with the rural problem in one state. Chapter 15 looks at the bottom line: were the initiatives effective in improving the recruitment and retention of physicians in the rural communities? Chapter 16 draws conclusions and makes pointed recommendations to various constituent groups who wish to duplicate or expand on the Arkansas experience.

In all candor there always will be a rural problem. The distribution of goods and the access to care inevitably will plague those who live and work far from urban centers. But there are solutions, good and acceptable alternatives, and our experience encourages us to be optimistic about the future options.

Chapter 15
Assessment of Rural Program Successes and Failures
by Thomas Allen Bruce, M.D.

The interdependence of actions in the several sectors of health service has become increasingly recognized as necessary for rural improvements. Programs for facility construction, manpower expansion, economic support, and quality promotion are all obviously intertwined. These actions, in turn, are all interdependent with general social changes in agriculture, employment, transportation, education, social security, and other spheres. Reaching goals in any one of these sectors usually depends on parallel actions in several of the others.

... Milton I. Roemer, 1976

This book obviously would not have been written had the rural practice program of the College of Medicine been a disaster. It was not a disaster, but it also has not been an unmitigated success. It is fortunate that what progress has been achieved has been highly visible. This chapter will attempt to evaluate the particular components of the program which were most worthwhile, and those which have turned out to be disappointing.

Physician recruitment and retention is a complex problem. It is not a matter of building a clinic. It is not a matter of hiring a recruiting agency. It is not guaranteeing a physician a certain annual income. These are stop-gap measures which are temporary at best. Physician recruitment and retention is tied into the very fabric of a community, with the interaction of many attributes which make up that community and contribute to its "wellness" or to its inability to solve local problems.

The best single achievement of the Rural Medical Development Program has been to establish a working relationship of the College with the state's needy communities; it has set up an organized consultation and technical assistance system that previously was not available from any source. The greatest gain has accrued to the College itself: its credibility, its public identity, its visible commitment to societal responsibility in the broad sense . . . the move away from simply educating doctors.

The state's communities clearly have benefited from the Program also. Previously isolated, working at serious disadvantage in not understanding the medical care "system," vulnerable to the latest recruiting gimmick and to a few unscrupulous individuals who took advantage of their lack of understanding, these communities have found the Medical College Program an available resource of willing help and a place of expertise in the complexities of the "matching" game. The Program has not just incidentally provided access to the new physicians coming out of the medical training programs.

Finally, the medical graduates have gained from the Program. The outreach activities and spectrum of opportunities to meet practicing physicians and community leaders outside the "pressurized" recruiting agency environment, the ability to have better front-end knowledge of the needs in maintaining a rural practice, and the counsel and professional assistance of the College staff inevitably have allowed for a more rational, logical approach to selecting a community for practice.

It is a basic consideration that the Rural Medical Development Program could have achieved one or both of the following: 1) improved recruitment of physicians to rural communities, and 2) improved retention of physicians in rural communities.

It is the considered judgment of the Program staff members after several years of work in this field that recruitment represents about 20% of the issue to be solved, and retention about 80%. The findings indicate that if all the communities who had recruited physicians over the past several years had been able to keep them practicing in the community, there would be no problem of access to rural medical care today. It has been the assumption that however much the Rural Office might be successful in bringing about some increase in physician recruitment, the work would be ineffectual if major gains were not made in retention. It also has been assumed that progress would have an additive or cumulative effect, i.e., that the better the retention in a town, the easier it would be to recruit

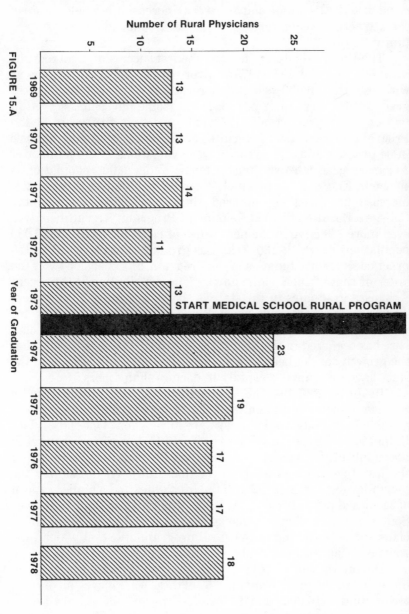

Recruitment of Arkansas Medical Graduates to Practice in Towns Smaller than 6,000 Population

Number of Rural Physicians

Year	Value
1969	13
1970	13
1971	14
1972	11
1973	13
1974	23
1975	19
1976	17
1977	17
1978	18

START MEDICAL SCHOOL RURAL PROGRAM

Year of Graduation

FIGURE 15.A

163

and retain additional physicians in that town because of the "critical numbers" phenomenon. Under that concept, the availability of new group practice options and of relief from the major disincentives in rural practice (isolation and overwork) increasingly would improve the attractiveness of rural practice as a bona fide career opportunity.

The Program has, in fact, had modest success in rural recruitment. During the 1969-1973 control period, the Arkansas towns with less than 6,000 population recruited 64 Arkansas medical graduates to serve in 72 practice sites (some physicians served in two or more practice sites). During the first five years of the Program the same towns recruited 85 Arkansas graduates to serve in 94 practice sites. The year by year variations in the number of Arkansas graduates settling in towns under 6,000 population is shown in Figure 15.A, in which it can be seen that an average 30% increase has been encountered since the inauguration of the College's Rural Medical Development Program. Recruitment was even more effective in the next order of rural towns (6,000-16,000 population) in which 130 Arkansas graduates have served in 150 practice sites since the start of the Program, an expansion twice the order of that of the smaller towns. The distribution of the recent Arkansas graduates in the state is shown in Figure 15.B. If non-Arkansas graduates who have elected to practice in the state are included, it can be seen that a sizable expansion of the physician base has occurred in five years (Figure 15.C). It also is evident that the growth has not been an even one, and that some sections of the state have grown more rapidly in doctors than others.

In June 1983 the U.S. Department of Health and Human Services issued a report entitled "Diffusion and the Changing Geographic Distribution of Primary Care Physicians." One of the tables in that report, reproduced here as Table 15.1, reported changes in the supply of office-based Primary Care Physicians by state during the last five years of analysis: in that study, Arkansas had the fourth-largest increase (22%) of the fifty states and a higher ratio of office-based primary care physicians to population than most other Southern states. This is in marked contrast to the number of physicians at the beginning of the rural program effort, at which time Arkansas had the most depleted supply of physicians in the nation.

During the control period of the study one graduate in every six moved from one town to another; 57 of these were moves out of rural towns (under 16,000) and 91 involved moves out of urban communities. Since 1974 only one graduate in every fifteen has moved from the community of initial practice, a much improved ratio of retention, but unfortunately two-thirds of these moves have

164

involved rural communities. Although progress has been achieved, the critical number of physicians in the rural communities has not been reached, and attrition even now remains all too high.

A great deal of the ultimate success in rural retention is dependent on the quality of the interlocking bond which unites the physician and the community. A properly educated physician who lands in a receptive and supportive community most often stays in that practice for a lifetime. Those efforts in the College of Medicine which have been most helpful in the development of that solid bond are, in the opinion of the staff:

1. Development of the Area Health Education Centers (AHECs).
2. Expansion of good primary care residency positions in the state.
3. Move of the Rural Preceptorship Program to an earlier position in the curriculum.
4. Development of the Office of Community Medical Affairs with its host of outreach and bridging activities.

Site of Practice, Recent Arkansas Medical Graduates, 1972-82

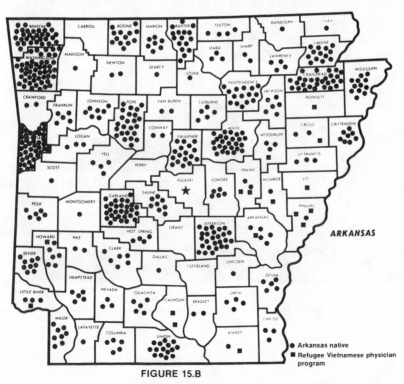

FIGURE 15.B

165

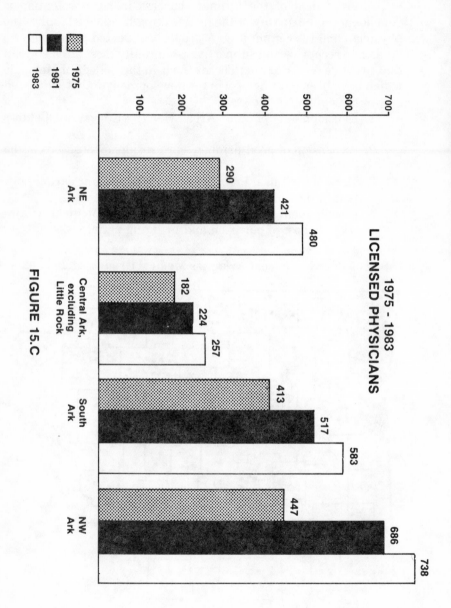

1975 - 1983
LICENSED PHYSICIANS

	1975	1981	1983
NE Ark	290	421	480
Central Ark, excluding Little Rock	182	224	257
South Ark	413	517	583
NW Ark	447	686	738

FIGURE 15.C

TABLE 15.1
Changes in the Supply of Office-based Primary Care M.D. and D.O. Physicians by State; 1975 to 1979

	Number of M.D. and D.O. Physicians		Ratio to Population		Percent Change in Ratio
	1975	1979	1975	1979	
Total	99,472	116,609	47	51	9
Alabama	1,080	1,280	30	33	10
Alaska	125	175	36	44	22
Arizona	1,274	1,677	57	62	9
Arkansas	729	906	34	40	18
California	11,593	13,721	55	58	5
Colorado	1,392	1,734	55	60	9
Connecticut	1,468	1,646	47	53	13
Delaware	254	298	44	50	14
District of Columbia	510	592	71	93	31
Florida	3,972	5,415	48	56	17
Georgia	1,690	1,980	34	36	6
Hawaii	418	560	48	58	21
Idaho	343	412	42	44	5
Illinois	4,800	5,528	43	48	12
Indiana	2,170	2,362	41	43	5
Iowa	1,365	1,633	48	56	17
Kansas	1,071	1,260	47	53	13
Kentucky	1,245	1,403	37	38	3
Louisiana	1,253	1,436	33	34	3
Maine	585	733	55	65	18
Maryland	1,722	2,073	42	49	17
Massachusetts	2,861	2,935	49	51	4
Michigan	5,296	6,271	58	68	17
Minnesota	1,873	2,179	48	53	10
Mississippi	723	861	31	34	10
Missouri	2,518	2,965	53	60	13
Montana	350	400	47	51	9
Nebraska	657	727	43	46	7
Nevada	235	325	40	41	3
New Hampshire	384	431	47	47	0
New Jersey	3,783	4,198	52	57	10
New Mexico	493	599	43	46	7
New York	9,557	9,622	53	55	4

167

TABLE 15.1 (continued)

	Number of M.D. and D.O. Physicians		Ratio to Population		Percent Change in Ratio
	1975	1979	1975	1979	
North Carolina	1,878	2,261	34	38	12
North Dakota	264	296	41	45	10
Ohio	5,077	5,839	47	54	15
Oklahoma	1,306	1,652	48	55	15
Oregon	1,231	1,510	54	57	6
Pennsylvania	6,397	7,460	54	63	17
Rhode Island	480	536	52	57	10
South Carolina	914	1,118	32	36	13
South Dakota	245	290	36	42	17
Tennessee	1,405	1,695	34	37	9
Texas	5,248	6,423	43	45	5
Utah	471	557	39	38	-3
Vermont	273	309	58	60	3
Virginia	1,854	2,945	37	45	22
Washington	1,816	2,205	51	53	4
West Virginia	665	762	37	39	5
Wisconsin	1,995	2,233	43	47	9
Wyoming	164	176	44	37	-16

The efforts which continue to be serious deterrents to rural medical practice are outlined below. None of the efforts in the College of Medicine have addressed these effectively.

1. Inadequate medical facilities and support systems (i.e., transportation) in the rural community.
2. Lack of career opportunities for spouse or educational opportunities for the children in the rural community.
3. Lack of opportunity for group practice and of professional liaison in the rural community, and
4. Economic disadvantages of practice in those rural communities in which poverty and unemployment are extremely high or in which the entire business and financial infrastructure fails to thrive.

To those medical schools who are planning to improve their efforts in rural development it is suggested that a broad-brush approach be used in which faculty, students and administrative officials equally are expected to participate in planning and implementing the program. There must be a serious and visible commitment from the medical school to make a contribution to rural medicine and to support the existing rural practitioners.

To those legislative groups who would like to expand the quality and quantity of health services in rural areas it is suggested that efforts be made to finance properly the regional educational centers, to sponsor those incentive programs for rural hospitals, clinics and professionals which have been carefully coordinated with the educational ventures, and to look at better ways in which government-subsidized health care can support, rather than undercut, rural medical care.

To those professional societies that would like to facilitate rural medical practice it is suggested that the complex problems of professional isolation be addressed, plus the need for continuing medical education and the need for special support systems to work with isolated instances of "problem" physicians who need help because of physical, mental, social or professional difficulties. The professional societies also could usefully set up practice management consulting groups that would be of considerable aid to their members, especially those newly entering practice.

To those rural communities who are looking for help, it is suggested that, while outside consultation, advice and technical and financial assistance can be most valuable, in the long run it will be up to the leadership within your own town to analyze collectively the special problems to be addressed, and to carry out a logical effort to solve those problems. And while it is recognized that leadership is ephemeral and changing, development of the proper leaders surely is within the reach of all those who wish to promote their own future well-being!

Chapter 16
Recommendations for Study and Action

Throughout this book an attempt has been made to draw conclusions from the rural studies and special initiatives which might have relevant medical or public policy implication. All of the results have been interesting and useful for what they reveal relative to the characteristics of practicing physicians. However, the results frequently have suggested that decisions on rural placement or retention issues reflect intrinsic personal and private values and motives where public policymakers are unlikely to have any impact. Some results do suggest areas where a new program or a new policy potentially could effect the retention of physicians or health professionals in the most needy areas. Some of these programmatic and policy implications have been mentioned in earlier chapters.

At the completion of the comprehensive study on Arkansas physicians carried out by the Research office, the Dean's staff reviewed the material in depth and at a group process planning retreat made some recommendations for futher action. The overriding concept under which the recommendations fall is the reversal of the trend which saw most medical graduates entering specialty and sub-specialty practice in larger cities. Let it be clear that there is nothing wrong about the concentration of significant numbers of medical and surgical specialists in regional centers to provide the latest technological advances in medical care. The priority needs in this and other states, however, now and in the future, undoubtedly lie in general (nonspecialized) medical and health care in the smaller towns and more rural areas. Specific conclusions of the group process deliberations were:

    I. Colleges of medicine should attempt to decrease the career impact of specialty and sub-specialty training on the educational process by a number of initiatives, some of which may be the following:

A. Strengthening the teaching emphasis on *general* medicine concepts and care in the junior year clinical clerkships

B. Increasing the teaching emphasis on ambulatory care, as opposed to hospital inpatient care, thus providing a closer correlation to the priorities of care which exist in rural areas.

C. Broadening the use of the multidisciplinary team-care approach in teaching medical students so that they learn by example and role model.

D. Expanding the rural preceptorships program to become part of the core medical school curriculum so as to increase medical student exposure to rural areas.

E. Increasing the exposure of medical students to the discipline of family practice through new clinical clerkships and additional preceptorship opportunities.

F. Increasing the number of family practice residency positions since those physicians are more likely to practice in rural areas.

G. Strengthening supportive services to physicians in rural practice to relieve isolation. Such supportive services might include additional consultation, for instance the increased utilization of telephone consultation efforts, and communication of other types, including the possibility of statewide or regional audiovisual communications networks.

H. Exploring additional opportunities for the medical faculty members to engage in locum tenens practice during vacation periods, in order to increase their understanding of rural practice needs.

I. Exploring the potential and the ramifications of free-standing rural practice residency programs.

J. Developing a major locus for rural health efforts including research, community development, and educational activities specifically oriented to the needs of rural health care.

II. Colleges of medicine should increase technical assistance to rural communities by:

A. Helping to develop alternative health care systems for problem areas.

B. Providing consultation relative to health facilities, planning and development.

C. Promoting the concept of *group* practice to rural com-

172

munities seeking physicians and to students looking for practice opportunities.

D. Creating more opportunities for student and house-staff interaction in community planning-development processes and improving their information relative to rural practice opportunities.

E. Exploring to determine the most effective techniques in counseling communities on their physician recruitment and retention problem, to include heavy emphasis on alternative systems for problem areas.

F. Exploring the potential of an early identification of problem communities and the possibility of intervention prior to the point where the problems become so severe that they do not lend themselves to solution.

III. Colleges of medicine should provide additional emphasis to admitting rural students to the medical education program by:

A. Expanding the program for recruiting a greater number of qualified rural students by looking particularly at early (high school and before) career counseling for minority and disadvantaged students from rural backgrounds.

B. Develop improved techniques for determining rural practice interest in those applying for admission.

IV. The Area Health Education Centers/Continuing Medical Education Programs should increase their role and relationships with communities and community physicians in order to reduce isolation in rural communities by:

A. Expanding the continuing medical education program to include a greater emphasis on courses offered throughout the state, thus providing better accessibility to rural physicians. The program should explore the extension of audiovisual communications in AHEC/ CME programs and the use of electronic media for long-distance teaching purposes.

B. Reinforcing the use of feedback from the telephone consultation system throughout the spectrum of medical education. Reorienting the individual AHECs toward specific geographic areas of the state in order that they may assume greater area responsibility.

V. Colleges of medicine should engage in additional research or exploration in rural health care by:

A. Conducting additional community research with emphasis on direct interviewing in the communities in

173

order to provide a fuller understanding of the dynamics of recruitment and retention from the community perspective.

B. Exploring the process of career decision-making in rural physicians in order than the phenomenon may be more fully understood.

C. Evaluating the implications of the "urbanization" of rural life.

VI. States with a commitment to upgrade the quality and availability of health care services should increase their involvement in rural health issues by:

A. Exploring the potential of regionalized rural health facilities and services, including primary, secondary and tertiary care access for each geographic region.

B. Expanding primary care facilities in rural areas.

C. Studying health payment systems to determine a better system for reimbursement for care of poverty, low income and disadvantaged citizens.

D. Increasing the supply of non-physician members of health professional teams to provide support for a rural physician and to extend the physician's capabilities.

E. Improving emergency transportation service resources for patients to regional medical centers.

APPENDIX
The Art of Teaching

By George L. Ackerman, M.D.
Professor of Medicine
University of Arkansas for Medical Sciences

Editor's note: Each volunteer physician in the Preceptorship program receives the following brief article by Dr. Ackerman, one of the outstanding master-teachers in the UAMS College of Medicine.

Teaching is an art, not a science, so that an approach to teaching that is effective for one person may not be for another. Some generalizations can be made, however.

The teacher himself, his personality, attitudes, and demeanor is as important in assuring successful teaching as the teaching method used. What are the qualities of a good teacher? Gilbert Highet in his book, *The Art of Teaching*, lists three:

1) He must know his subject.
2) He must like his subject, and like teaching it.
3) He must like his students.

To these I would add, and this is especially important for rural preceptors, that he must be willing to grant the *time* required for teaching. Further, one would hope that the teacher knew more than just his subject—that he served as a bridge between his subject and the world. The teaching method most commonly used in clinical instruction is the tutorial technique, and the refinement on it that may be called the Socratic method. Teaching this way is expensive in time and effort, but is a very effective and rewarding way of teaching. In this form of teaching, the student is led from the simple to the complex with carefully chosen questions and responses to his answers.

This method:
1) Insures student participation.
2) Allows the teacher to know what the student has grasped and his areas of uncertainty.
3) Illustrates the "logic of medicine", i.e. the flow from the simple to the complex.
4) Forces the student to formulate his ideas and concepts.

What a teacher says outright sometimes goes unheard. What he stimulates his pupils to think out for themselves often has a far more potent influence on them.

The preceptorship is a somewhat special teaching situation. Some of my thoughts on this experience are:
1) To be a purely passive observer soon becomes boring. The student must be involved in your activities.
2) The student must be given some responsibility; ideally this should increase during his time with you.
3) Let the student teach you. Ask questions and encourage him to share what he has learned.
4) Try to demonstrate the value of his prior educational experiences. Be a link between medical school and medical practice.
5) Praise is a valued reward and a potent stimulus to further efforts. Certainly correct mistakes, but remember to recognize good work.
6) Assuming the role of a teacher—joining a university faculty—is not a light responsibility. A respect for learning, an open mind that is tolerant of new ideas and skeptical of dogma, willingness to admit mistakes, and finally the knack of not taking one's self too seriously should be the marks of the educated man.

Rural Preceptorship: Educational Objectives

The student will have the opportunity to observe, and be a part of, all aspects of the practice of primary care medicine in a small community. In so doing, he will gain knowledge and develop basic skills in dealing with common health problems in that community.

Knowledge—The student will learn:
1) the types of medical problems commonly seen by the private practitioner
2) the natural course of these problems
3) the techniques commonly applied for the prevention, diagnosis, and treatment of these problems

4) the human interactions in the patient's immediate environment (family and community) which are important in dealing with these problems
5) the community and state resources available which relate to health
6) the basic principles of good office management

Skills—the student will develop basic skills in:
1) an approach to clinical problem recognition
2) the maintenance of good clinical records
3) conducting patient interviews
4) performing simple diagnostic and therapeutic procedures

Selected References on
Rural Health

Ahearn, Mary C. *Health Care in Rural America.* U.S. Department of Agriculture Bulletin No. 428, Washington, D.C., 1979.

Anderson, James G. and Bartkus, David E. "Physician Location and Distribution: A Social Systems Approach," *Socio-Economic Planning Sciences* 10:213-221, 1976.

Area Health Education Centers: A Directory of Federal, State, Local and Private Decentralized Health Professional Education Programs: DHEW Publ., Hyattsville, Md. 1976.

Area Health Education Centers: A Directory of Federal, State, Local and Private Decentralized Health Professional Education Programs: Supplement. DHEW Publ. Hyattsville, Md., 1976.

Bachrach, Leona L., ed. *Human Services in Rural Areas.* Project Share, Rockville, Md., 1981.

Barton, S. N., ed. *Rural Health and Health Communication.* S. Karger Publ. Co., New York, 1977.

Beck, James D. and Gernert, Edward B. "Attitudes and Background Values as Predictors of Urban/Rural Practice Location," *Journal of Dental Education,* September 1971, pp. 573-81.

Bernstein, James D., Hege, Fredrick P. and Farran, Christopher C. *Rural Health Centers in the United States.* Ballinger Publ. Co., Cambridge, Mass., 1979.

Bible, Bond L. "Physicians' Views of Medical Practice in Nonmetropolitan Communities," *Public Health Reports* 85:1117, 1970.

Bisbee, Gerald E., Jr., ed. *Management of Rural Primary Care—Concepts and Cases.* Hospital Research and Educational Trust, Chicago, 1982.

Brooks, Edward F. and Wade, Torlen L., eds. *Planning and Managing Rural Health Centers*. Ballinger Publ. Co., Cambridge, Mass., 1979.

Bruce, Thomas A. "The Medical School, 1974-75," *Journal of the Arkansas Medical Society* 71:367-370, 1975.

Bruce, Thomas A. "University of Arkansas College of Medicine, 1975-76. Report of the 97th Year," *Journal of the Arkansas Medical Society* 73:265-270, 1976.

Bruce, Thomas A. "The Clinical Preceptorship in Medical Education," chapter in *Macy Conference Report on the Changing Medical Curriculum*. Josiah Macy, Jr. Foundation., New York, 1972.

Bruce, Thomas A. "The State of the College, University of Arkansas College of Medicine, 1980." *Journal of the Arkansas Medical Society* 78:93-96, 1981.

Bruce, Thomas A. "The College of Medicine in 1983: Pride and Concern" (editorial), *Journal of the Arkansas Medical Society* 79:455-56, 1983.

Bruhn, John G. and Parsons, Oscar A. "Attitudes Toward Medical Specialties: Two Follow-Up Studies," *Journal of Medical Education* 40:273-280, 1965.

Cantwell, James R. and Eisenberg, Barry S. *The Spatial Distribution of Physicians: A Literature Review*. AMA Center for Health Services Research and Development, June 1975.

Childs, Alan W. and Melton, Gary B., eds. *Rural Psychology*. Plenium Press, New York, 1982.

Coker, Robert E., Back, Kurt W., Donnelly, Thomas G. and Miller, Norman. "Patterns of Influence: Medical School Faculty Members and the Values and Specialty Interests of Medical Students," *Journal of Medical Education* 35:518-527, 1960.

Coker, Robert E., Miller, Norman, Back, Kurt W. and Donnelly, Thomas. "The Medical Student, Specialization and General Practice," *North Carolina Medical Journal* 21:96-101, 1960.

Coleman, Sinclair. *Physician Distribution and Access to Medical Services*, RAND, Santa Monica, April 1976. R-1887-HEW.

Cooper, James K., Heald, Karen and Samuels, Michael, "Affecting the Supply of Rural Physicians," *American Journal of Public Health* 67:756-759, 1977.

Cooper, James K., Heald, Karen and Samuels, Michael, "The Decision for Rural Practice," *Journal of Medical Education* 47:939-944, 1972.

Cordes, Sam M. *Rural Health Care Delivery: A Compilation of Recent and Ongoing Research.* Agricultural Economics and Rural Sociology Publ. 163, Penn. State University, University Park, PA, 1983.

Cordes, Sam M. and Barkley, Paul W. *Physicians and Physician Services in Rural Washington.* Bulletin 790, Washington Agricultural Experiment Station, January 1974.

Couto, Richard A. *Streams of Idealism and Health Care Innovation: An Assessment of Service-Learning and Community Mobilization.* Teachers College, Columbia University, New York, 1982.

Crawford, Ronald L. and McCormack, Regina C. "Reasons Physicians Leave Primary Practice," *Journal of Medical Education* 46:263-268, 1971.

Cullison, Sam. *Literature Review and Critical State-of-Art Survey: Physician Location and Specialty Choice.* AMA Center for Health Services Research and Development, February 1975.

Cullison, Sam, Reid, Christopher and Colwill, Jack. "Medical School Admissions, Specialty Selection, and Distribution of Physicians," *JAMA* 235:502-505, 1976.

Decentralization and Regionalization of Health Professional Education and Training: Proceedings of the National Conference, April 25-27, 1975. DHEW Publ., Hyattsville, Md., 1975.

Delivery of Health Care in Rural America. American Hospital Association, 1977.

DeVise, Pierre. "Physician Migration from Inland to Coastal States: Antipodal Examples of Illinois and California," *Journal of Medical Education* 48:141-151, 1973.

DeVries, Robert A. and Cleary, Joan L. "Rural Health Care at the Crossroad," *American Rural Health Newsletter* 2:3-4, 1983.

Directory of Rural Health Care Programs. U.S. Dept. of Health, Education, and Welfare, Washington, D.C., 1979.

Diseker, Robert A. and Chappell, James A. "Relative Importance of Variables in Determination of Practice Location: A Pilot Study," *Social Science and Medicine* 10:559-563, 1976.

Doermann, A. C. and others. *Selected Approaches to Enhancing the Retention of Primary Care Physicians in Rural Practice.* The Mitre Corporation, McLean, Va., 1975.

Donofrio, Carol and Wang, Virginia, eds. *Cooperative Rural Health Education.* Slack, Inc., Thorofare, N.J., 1976.

Donovan, John C., Salzman, Leonard F. and Allen, Peter Z. "Studies in Medical Education: The Role of Cognitive and Psychological Characteristics as Career Choice Correlates," *American Journal of Obstetrics and Gynecology* 114:461-467, 1972.

Evashwick, Connie J. "The Role of Group Practice in the Distribution of Physicians in Nonmetropolitan Areas," *Medical Care* 14:808-823, 1976.

Fahs, Ivan J. and Peterson, Osler L. "Towns Without Physicians and Towns With Only One—A Study of Four States in the Upper Midwest," 1965, *American Journal of Public Health* 58:1200-1211, 1968.

Fein, Rashi and Weber, Gerald I. *Financing Medical Education.* McGraw Hill, New York, 1971.

Fields, Cheryl M. "Educators Doubt Doctors Will Stay in Remote Areas," *Chronicle of Higher Education*, October 25, 1976.

Fishman, Daniel B. and Zimet, Carl N. "Specialty Choice and Beliefs About Specialties Among Freshman Medical Students," *Journal of Medical Education* 47:524-533, 1972.

Freshley, Harold B. "Change in Medical Students' Perceptions of Practicing Medicine in Small Communities," Section of Behavioral Sciences Course, University of Missouri-Columbia Medical School, 1977.

Geertsma, Robert H. and Grinols, Donald R. "Specialty Choice in Medicine," *Journal of Medical Education* 47:509-517, 1972.

Gough, Harrison G. "Specialty Preferences of Physicians and Medical Students," *Journal of Medical Education* 50:581-588, 1975.

Hassinger, Edward W. and Whiting, Larry, eds. *Rural Health Services: Organization, Delivery and Use.* Iowa State University Press, Ames, 1982.

Hassinger, Edward W. *Rural Health Organization: Social Networks and Regionalization.* Iowa State University Press, Ames, 1982.

Heald, Karen A. and Cooper, James K. *An Annotated Bibliography on Rural Medical Care.* RAND, Santa Monica, April 1972, R-966-HEW.

Heald, Karen A., Cooper, James K. and Coleman, Sinclair. *Choice of Location of Practice of Medical School Graduates: Analysis of Two Surveys.* RAND, Santa Monica, November 1974, R-1477-HEW.

Health Professionals for the South: Supply and Cost Issues Needing State Attention. Report of the Southern Regional Education Board, Atlanta, 1983.

182

Health Professional Manpower Shortage Area Plan: Final Report and Appendices, University of Texas Health Science Center, Houston, February 1975.

Henderson, William and Elliott, Katherine. *More Technologies for Rural Health.* Scholium International, Inc., Great Neck, N.Y., 1980.

Herman, Mary W. and Veloski, Jon. "Family Medicine and Primary Care: Trends and Student Characteristics," *Journal of Medical Education* 52:99-106, 1977.

Hough, Douglas E. and Marder, William D. "State Retention of Medical School Graduates," *Journal of Medical Education.* 57:505-513, 1982.

Johnson, H. Wayne, ed. *Rural Human Services.* Peacock, Itasca, Ill., 1980.

Johnson, Vardell, Norton, W. Richard and Bruce, Thomas A. "Factors Influencing Medical Student and Housestaff Specialty Choice and Planned Practice Location," *American Journal of Rural Health* 5:1-14, 1980.

Joroff, Sheila and Navarro, Vincente. "Medical Manpower: A Multi-Variate Analysis of the Distribution of Physicians in Urban United States," *Medical Care* 9:428-438, 1971.

Kane, Robert L. and others. "Mail-Order Medicine: An Analysis of the Sears Roebuck Foundation's Community Medical Assistance Program," *JAMA* 232:1023-1027, 1975.

Kaufman, Mark. "How to Influence Physicians' Decisions for Rural Practice," *Journal of the Maine Medical Association* 63:276-279, 1976.

Kegel-Flom, Penelope. "Predictors of Rural Practice Location," *Journal of Medical Education* 52:204-209, 1977.

Korman, Louis and Feldman, Harry A. "A Study of the Recruitment of Physicians into Three Northern New York Counties," *Journal of Medical Education* 52:308-315, 1977.

Krans, A. S., Botterell, E. H., Einarson, D. W. and Thompson, M. G. "Initial Career Plans and Subsequent Family Practice," *Journal of Medical Education* 46:826-830, 1971.

Liccione, William J. and McAllister, Susan. "Attitudes of First-Year Medical Students Toward Rural Medical Practice," *Journal of Medical Education* 49:449-451, 1974.

Longnecker, Douglas P. "Practice Objectives and Goals: A Survey of Family Practice Residents," *Journal of Family Practice* 2:347-351, 1975.

Lucas, Rex A. and Himelfarb, Alexander. "Some Social Aspects of Medical Care in Small Communities," *Canadian Journal of Public Health* 62:6-16, 1971.

MacNair, Ray. *Community Partnership Organizations: A Better Way to Gain Participation in Health Programs.* U.S.P.H.S. Centers for Disease Control, Atlanta, 1980.

Madison, Donald L. *Starting Out in Rural Practice.* University of North Carolina, Chapel Hill, 1980.

Madison, Donald L. "Recruiting Physicians for Rural Practice," *Health Services Reports* 88:758-762, 1973.

Madison, Donald L. and Bernstein, James D. "Rural Health Care and the Rural Hospital." *Community Hospital and Primary Care* by Bryant, John H. and others. Ballinger, Cambridge, 1976.

Marden, Parker G. "A Demographic and Ecological Analysis of the Distribution of Physicians in Metropolitan America, 1960," *American Journal of Sociology* 72:290-300, 1966.

Marshall, Carter L. and others. "Principal Components Analysis of the Distribution of Physicians, Dentists, and Osteopaths in a Midwestern State," *American Journal of Public Health* 63:1556-1562, 1971.

Martin, Edward D., Moffat, Robert E., Falter, Richard T. and Walker, Jack D. "The University of Kansas School of Medicine: A Study of The Profile of 959 Graduates and Factors Which Influenced the Geographic Distribution," *Journal of the Kansas Medical Society* 69:84-89, 1968.

Mason, Henry R. "Medical School, Residency, and Eventual Practice Location," *JAMA* 233:49-52, 1975.

Matteson, Michael T. and Smith, Samuel V. "Selection of Medical Specialties: Preferences Versus Choices," *Journal of Medical Education* 52:548-554, 1977.

McConnell, Diane C., Kohls, James M., Norton, W. Richard and Bruce, Thomas A. "Factors Influencing Physician Recruitment and Retention in Two Types of Rural Communities," *American Journal of Rural Health* 5:19-32, 1980.

McFarland, John. "Toward an Explanation of the Geographical Location of Physicians in the United States," *Measuring Physician Manpower*, AMA Center for Health Sciences Research and Development, 1973. pp. 17-38.

McGrath, Ellen and Zimet, Carl N. "Female and Male Medical Students: Differences in Specialty Choice Selection and Personality," *Journal of Medical Education* 52:293-300, 1977.

McNerney, Walter J. and Riedel, Donald C., eds. *Regionalization and Rural Health Care, An Experiment in Three Communities.* University of Michigan Press, Ann Arbor, 1978.

Mountin, Joseph, Pennell, E. H. and Nicolay, Virginia. "Location and Movement of Physicians, 1923 and 1938: Effect of Local Factors Upon Location," *Public Health Reports* 57:1945-1954, 1942.

Mullner, Ross and O'Rouke, Thomas. "A Geographic Analysis of Counties Without an Active Non-Federal Physician, United States, 1963-71," *Health Services Reports* 89:256-262, 1974.

Mustian, R. David. *Rural Health Care: A Bibliography.* Southern Rural Development Center, Mississippi State, MS, 1980.

Norton, W. Richard, Culp, William L. and Bruce, Thomas A. "Geographic Distribution of 1962-71 Graduates of University of Arkansas College of Medicine," *Journal of the Arkansas Medical Scoiety* 74:151-155, 1977.

Norton, W. Richard, Jackson, John S., McConnell, Diane C., Jackson, Judith A. and Bruce, Thomas A. *Recruitment and Retention of Physicians in Rural Arkansas.* Report to the Winthrop Rockefeller Foundation, Little Rock, 1978.

Oates, Richard P. and Feldman, Harry A. "Patterns of Change in Medical Student Career Choices," *Journal of Medical Education* 49:562-569, 1974.

Oates, Richard P. and Feldman, Harry A. "Medical Career Patterns: Choices Among Several Classes of Medical Students," *New York State Journal of Medicine* 71:2437-2440, 1971.

O'Connor, R. W. *Managing Health Systems in Developing Areas.* Lexington Book Co., Lexington, Mass., 1980.

Odegaard, Charles E. *Eleven Area Health Education Centers. The View From the Grass Roots.* Carnegie Council Policy, University of Washington Press, Seattle, 1980.

Odegaard, Charles E. *Area Health Education Centers. The Pioneering Years, 1972-1978.* University of Washington Press, Seattle, 1980.

O'Leary, Jean A. and O'Leary, John B. "Community Development and Rural Health: Costa Rica and Minnesota," *American Journal of Rural Health* 5:15-17, 1980.

Parker, R. C. and Tuxill, T. G. "The Attitude of Physicians Toward Small Community Practice," *Journal of Medical Education* 42:327-344, 1967.

Parker, R. C., Rix, R. A. and Tuxill, T. G. "Social, Economic and Demographic Factors Affecting Physician Population in Upstate New York," *New York State Journal of Medicine* 69: 706-712, 1969.

Pavia, Rosalia E. A. and Haley, Harold B. "Intellectual, Personality, and Environmental Factors in Career Specialty Preferences," *Journal of Medical Education* 46:281-289, 1971.

Perlstadt, Harry. "Internship Placements and Faculty Influence," *Journal of Medical Education* 47:862-868, 1972.

Peterson, Gary R. "A Comparison of Selected Professional and Social Characteristics of Urban and Rural Physicians in Iowa," University of Iowa Health Care Research Series No. 8, 1968.

Plovnick, Mark. "Primary Care Career Choices and Medical Student Learning Styles," *Journal of Medical Education* 50:849-855, 1975.

Project Hope. *Urban and Rural Health Care in the Americas.* Hope Press, Millwood, Va., 1980.

Rakel, Robert E. "A Better Break for the Rural Physician," *Prism* 1:56-66, 1973.

Report of the Secretary, DHEW, *An Assessment of the National Area Health Education Center Program.* DHEW Publ., Hyattsville, Md., 1980.

Retention of National Health Service Corps Physicians in Health Manpower Shortage Areas. Family Health Care., Inc., February 1, 1977. HRA-DHEW No. 282-76-0439.

Rimlinger, Gaston V. and Steele, Henry B. "An Economic Interpretation of the Spatial Distribution of Physicians in the U.S.," *Southern Economics Journal* 30:1-12, 1963.

Roemer, Milton I. *Rural Health Care.* C. V. Mosby Co., St. Louis, 1976.

Rosenblatt, Roger A. and Moscovice, Ira S. *Rural Health Care.* John Wiley and Sons, New York, 1982.

Rourke, Anthony J. J. "Small Town Doctor Needs More Than An Office," *Modern Hospital* 117:151, 1971.

Rural Health: A Study and Plan for Expanding Primary Care Services in North-East Central Texas. University of Texas Health Science Center (Dallas), August 1975.

Rushing, William A. "Public Policy, Community Constraints, and the Distribution of Medical Resources," *Social Problems* 19:21-36, 1971.

Rushing, William A. and Wade, George T. "Community-Structure Constraints on Distribution of Physicians," *Health Services Research* 8:283-397, 1973.

Rushing, William A. *Community, Physicians, and Inequality.* D.C. Heath and Co., Lexington, Mass., 1975.

Schroeder, Steven A. and Schliftman, Alan. "The Influence of Medical School on Selection of Career Specialties," *Medical Annals of the District of Columbia* 42:339-343, 1973.

Schwartz, Lawrence E. and Cantwell, James R. "Weiskotten Survey, Class of 1960: A Profile of Physician Location and Specialty Choice," *Journal of Medical Education* 51:533-540, 1976.

Shannon, Robert. "National Health Service Corps: Overview and New Directions." Report of the Regional Workshops on Health Manpower Distribution, National Health Council, New York, 1975.

Sivertson, S. E. and Meyer, T. C. "Student Evaluation of Medical Preceptorships," *Wisconsin Medical Journal* 70:39-41, 1971.

Steele, Henry B. and Rimlinger, Gaston V. "Income Opportunities and Physician Location Trends in the United States," *Western Economics Journal* 3:182-194, 1967.

Steinwald, Bruce and Steinwald, Carolyn. "The Effect of Preceptorship and Rural Training Programs on Physicians' Practice Location Decision," *Medical Care* 13:219-229, 1975.

Taylor, Mark, Dickman, William and Kane, Robert. "Medical Students' Attitudes Toward Rural Practice," *Journal of Medical Education* 48:885-895, 1973.

Tyrell, D. A., Burkitt, D. P. and Henderson, William. *Technologies for Rural Health.* Royal Society of London Publications, Scholium International, Inc., Great Neck, N.Y., 1978.

U.S. Bureau of the Census, *U.S. Census of Population: 1970, Number of Inhabitants.* U.S. Government Printing Office, Washington, 1971.

U.S. Senate, Hearing before the Special Committee on Aging. "Rural Health Care for the Elderly: New Paths for the Future." U.S. Government Printing Office, Washington, D.C., 1982.

Varner, Melba S. and McCandless, Amy M., eds. "Proceedings of a Symposium on Culture and Health: Implications for Health Policy in Rural South Carolina." College of Charleston, South Carolina, 1979.

Voth, Donald E. "An Evaluation of Community Development Programs in Illinois," *Social Forces* 53:635-646, 1975.

Wallack, Stanley S. and Kretz, Sandra E. *Rural Medicine: Obstacles and Solutions for Self-Sufficiency.* Lexington Books, Lexington, Mass., 1981.

Warren, David G. *A Legal Guide for Rural Health Programs.* Ballinger Publ. Co., Cambridge, Mass., 1979.

Warren, Roland L. "Toward a Non-Utopian Normative Model of the Community," *American Social Review* 35:219-228, 1970.

Wasserman, Edward, Yufit, Robert I. and Pollock, George H. "Medical Specialty Choice and Personality," *Archives of General Psychiatry* 21:529-535, 1969.